Population Genetics with R

Population Genetics with R

An Introduction for Life Scientists

ÁKI J. LÁRUSON
& FLOYD A. REED

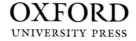

OXFORD
UNIVERSITY PRESS

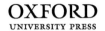

OXFORD
UNIVERSITY PRESS

Great Clarendon Street, Oxford OX2 6DP,
United Kingdom

Oxford University Press is a department of the University of Oxford.
It furthers the University's objective of excellence in research, scholarship,
and education by publishing worldwide. Oxford is a registered trade mark of
Oxford University Press in the UK and in certain other countries

© Áki J. Láruson and Floyd A. Reed 2021

The moral rights of the authors have been asserted

First Edition published in 2021

Impression: 1

Published in the United States of America by Oxford University Press
198 Madison Avenue, New York, NY 10016, United States of America

British Library Cataloguing in Publication Data

Data available

Library of Congress Control Number: 2020946917

ISBN 978–0–19–882953–9 (hbk.)
ISBN 978–0–19–882954–6 (pbk.)

DOI: 10.1093/oso/9780198829539.001.001

Printed and bound by
CPI Group (UK) Ltd, Croydon, CR0 4YY

Links to third party websites are provided by Oxford in good faith and
for information only. Oxford disclaims any responsibility for the materials
contained in any third party website referenced in this work.

Acknowledgements

The authors would like to thank Victoria Sindorf and Vanessa Reed for their patience, support, and help in writing this book, and our families and friends, near and far, whose support means more than they'll ever know. We would also like to thank Daniel Whitaker, Maria Costantini, Michael Wallstrom, Helen Sung, Justin Walguarnery, Molly Albecker, Sara Schaal, Alan Downey-Wall, Ffion Titmuss, Thais Bittar, and many graduate students at U. H. Mānoa for testing sections, finding errors, and providing feedback. Special thanks to Katie Lotterhos, who had to put up with this book taking up entirely too much time.

Thanks also to Ian Sherman and Charles Bath at OUP; their good nature and patience throughout this process has been remarkable, and special acknowledgments to Jolene Sutton, Jarosław Bryk, and Mohamed Noor for their help at various points along the road. Finally, the authors thank Charles Aquadro, Richard Harrison, Alex Kondrashov, Richard Durrett, Rasmus Nielsen, and many others for teaching fundamental aspects of population genetics.

Contents

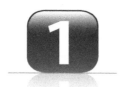

Learning through Programming

⊢ Term Definitions ⊢

Argument: A variable that is input into a function in a computer program.

Command Line Interface (CLI): A computer display window where a user can interface with the computer through text-based commands (sometimes called a terminal).

Function: A section of computer programming code that uses arguments as an input, completes a set of operations with those arguments, then outputs a result.

Graphical User Interface (GUI): A display where the user can interface with graphic icons using a cursor to make selections and issue commands.

Heuristic: A method of learning through direct practical implementation, which is not necessarily the most efficient.

Operating System: The software on a computer that serves as an interface between the computer's hardware and other software programs. Windows, Mac, and Linux are examples of operating systems.

1.1 Introduction

Population genetics, as a field of study, provides many important tools for scientists working with natural systems. It can be a conceptually challenging discipline, since it does not generally keep track of the individual organisms we might be studying, like a blue whale or a pine tree, or the outcomes of specific breeding events, in contrast to classical genetics.

Population Genetics with R: An Introduction for Life Scientists. Áki J. Láruson and Floyd A. Reed,
Oxford University Press (2021). © Áki J. Láruson & Floyd A. Reed.
DOI: 10.1093/oso/9780198829539.003.0001

Instead, population genetics seeks to determine the fundamental dynamics of genetic variation across an entire population, or even multiple populations, over the course of many generations. We can talk about changes in the frequency of specific genetic variants over time without keeping track of exactly which specific individuals do or do not have a particular copy of a variant. The famed quantitative biologist R. A. Fisher made a comparison between population genetics and the theory of gases in physics:

> The whole investigation may be compared to the analytical treatment of the Theory of Gases, in which it is possible to make the most varied assumptions as to the accidental circumstances, and even the essential nature of the individual molecules, and yet to develop the general laws as to the behaviour of gases, leaving but a few fundamental constants to be determined by experiment.
>
> (Fisher 1922).

Essentially one can predict a relationship between the pressure, volume, and temperature of a gas much like one can predict relationships between group size, inbreeding, and migration between populations, without keeping track of the specific interactions of all the individual molecules. The individual interactions give rise to overall emergent properties of the system.

This approach to biological questions is a bit abstract and can be difficult for new students to visualize. The visualization and study of the dynamics of genetic elements within and between populations requires a quantitative approach. An unfortunate side effect of the widespread implementation of ready-to-use quantitative software packages is that some facets of analysis can become rote, which at best might be implemented without the full understanding of the executor and at worst are applied inappropriately, leading to misguided conclusions. As quantitative models and methods become established in certain fields, it becomes necessary for people just entering a discipline to understand the thinking that goes into these approaches, so as to correctly interpret the results. In this book we aim to emphasize building an understanding of population genetics starting from fundamental principles. This book is *not* a guide to current software packages that can be used to carry out data processing in a "canned" way.

Learning anything requires dedication. Whether we are aware of it or not, we are investing an exceptional amount of ourselves when we learn something new. It could be something as willful as studying a new language, or something as innocuous as memorizing movie quotes. What we remember and what we forget from an experience can sometimes surprise us, and it is the perspective of the authors that "learning by doing" is especially true for the quantitative approaches necessary to really understand the field of population genetics. The challenge facing anyone wishing to learn population genetics methodologies is that it can be prohibitively laborious to calculate by hand the many parameters and summary statistics that lie at the heart of conceptual understanding. Fortunately, there exist a great many computer programs that allow for dataset manipulation and the implementation of these quantitative approaches.

Of particular note is the analytical software R, which has increasingly been the program of choice for exposure to basic statistical programming, as it is easily accessible (it's free!), has cross-platform compatibility (Windows, Mac, and Linux all support distributions of R), and has the potential of hands-on implementation by the reader as well as using pre-packaged implementation by the educator (such as readily shareable function definitions). R can be used purely as a CLI, but also has the option of well-supported free-to-use GUIs, such as RStudio (more on that later).

In this book we employ a series of heuristic approaches to help the reader develop an understanding of patterns and expectations in population genetics. We make the disclaimer that we are approaching the coding in a way that highlights specific concepts and therefore frequently implement code in a way that may seem cumbersome and inelegant to experienced programmers. There are many ways the code we present could be streamlined, but it is our hope that the structured way in which we present the code underscores the basic functional mechanisms involved as well as the population genetic concepts being addressed, and sets the reader up to move toward "leaner" and more efficient implementation later on in the book, as the expectation for both conceptual understanding and coding proficiency grows.

We urge readers to think about learning population genetics as an iterative process, as represented below, with the particular order of steps varying depending on which concept is being developed:

1. Start with logical arguments which can be written down as a model of a process.
2. Codify this model in a simple computer program to simulate the process and build a more intuitive understanding of the dynamics.
3. See how well the model predicts real data.
4. Use data to infer parameter values of the model.
5. Going back to step one, compare the original logical arguments and inference from data to refine the model.

At a higher level, we should start to see re-occurring patterns and interactions between different processes, for example, mutation, migration, drift, selection, etc., which should hopefully feed into a broader understanding of how these processes all contribute to the genetic make up of populations.

This book is not an exhaustive treatment of population genetics, statistics, and programming. These are rich and extensive fields and this book is intended as an introduction to point the way, *via ferrata*, to begin learning about these subjects so you don't have to start from scratch. The original literature is the best source of fundamental knowledge; however, it can be very cryptic and hard to follow at times. There are other textbooks that we highly recommend to continue learning and expanding your knowledge of population genetics. The full references for these textbooks are provided at the end of the book, but we want to highlight a select few here:

- Hartl and Clark (2006). This has served as a standard workhorse textbook of population genetics for many years.
- Gillespie (2004). This is a good resource for succinct additional theoretical background details about a range of population genetics topics.

- Slatkin and Nielsen (2013). This is another succinct guide that focuses on population genetics from a unifying perspective of the coalescent.
- Hedrick (2010). Like Hartl and Clark (2006), this goes into extensive details about a wide range of population genetics topics.

Ultimately, however, you will want to spend the time working through the original literature on subjects of interest to gain a fuller understanding.

1.2 Organization

We have tried to be consistent with some visual cues throughout this book. When referring to file names, object names, or names of buttons on the keyboard, we'll use `teletype` font to avoid confusion. We will color code different elements of the code; for example, when we talk about *functions* we will highlight them with a nice orange, while *arguments* within functions will be colored blue. As an example, the basic structure of a function will be represented like this: `function(argument = value)`. When we want to represent explicit code input and output, we'll use a box around the commands like this:

```
> print("Hello world!")
[1] "Hello world!"

> seq(from = 1, to = 7, by = 2) # We'll cover this
  soon!
[1] 1 3 5 7
```

As our code boxes get longer and more complex, we'll often want to include helpful comments in our code (which we'll color green) to help orient us and explain what is being done in different sections. To make comments inside your R code, just type "#" at the start of your comment and then R will ignore it!

Notice the greater-than signs ">" and the "[1]" symbols in the above box? Whenever you type commands into the R terminal the line of input automatically starts with a ">" symbol. So there's no need to type ">" at the beginning of your input code—it shows up automatically and signals the beginning of a new line of code. Similarly, the "[1]" shows up automatically whenever you have output from a code. In the example case above, we have one element that's output, so it's numbered as "[1]." If we had multiple elements of output from an input code, we would see each new element that's output numbered sequentially (for example, [1], [2], [3], …etc.).

But we're getting ahead of ourselves. In the next chapter we'll go through a brief background of the R language, and then go through actually finding and installing R on our computer.

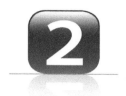

Downloading and Installing R

---| **Term Definitions** |---

Comprehensive R Archive Network (CRAN): An online repository of the R base system and contributed packages.

General Public License (GPL): A copyright agreement that allows for the free use, modification, and sharing of a software with the caveat that derivative work has to follow the same license.

GNU's Not Unix (GNU): An operating system and collection of software freely available through a GPL.

Gnu: Bovids native to Africa in the antelope genus *Connochaetes sp.*, also called wildebeest.

Hypertext Markup Language (HTML): A language commonly used to build web pages.

Interpreter: A computer program that executes (that is, implements) commands given in a specific programming language.

Package: A bundle of code, datasets, and documentation that is readily shareable between R users.

Script: A body of text containing pre-written code that can be executed all at once as a program.

Population Genetics with R: An Introduction for Life Scientists. Áki J. Láruson and Floyd A. Reed, Oxford University Press (2021). © Áki J. Láruson & Floyd A. Reed.
DOI: 10.1093/oso/9780198829539.003.0002

2.1 Introduction to R

The R statistical programming language has rapidly become the language of choice not just for introductory statistics courses, but also as a beginning language for people wanting to learn programming. While there are many other languages that may be better suited for general programming (such as Python, Perl, C++, Ruby, and some would even say Java), R has distinguished itself by being generally focused on dataset management and analysis, allowing neophytes to perform basic tasks relatively quickly.

Back in the early nineties, Drs. Ross Ihaka and Robert Gentleman at the University of Auckland, New Zealand, developed an interpreter (written in C) to support statistical programming work. Since both Dr. Ihaka and Dr. Gentleman were familiar with the Bell Laboratory programming language S, this new statistical language took on a similar syntax to S. In part as an acknowledgment of the influence of S and in part based on the first name initials of the two developers, this new language was dubbed R (Ihaka 1998, Hornik 2017). R was first distributed as an open-source software project with a GPL in 1995, and then in 2000 the stable distribution of R version 1.0.0 was released. Since then, R has become especially popular among researchers and academics.

One of R's big strengths as a language has been its dedicated and growing user community. Between online message boards where users help each other solve problems and user-developed packages containing unique scripts that are readily available through the CRAN (`https://cran.r-project.org/`), the R community is undoubtedly a major reason for the rapid adoption of this language by early learners. As of this writing, R is now in version 4.0.3 came out this last October, with millions of users worldwide and thousands of user-developed packages.

So how to get started? Well, another great thing about R is how easily available it is. It does require basic computer hardware and a working internet connection, but if you're using a Windows, Mac, or Linux operating system, installing R should be quick and painless. The first step is to go to the CRAN website (`https://cran.r-project.org/`, see

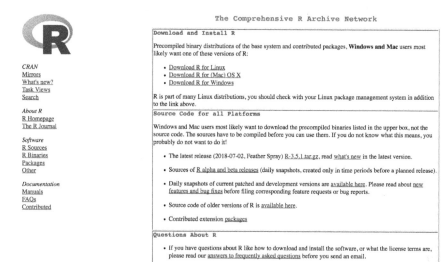

Figure 2.1 The front page of the Comprehensive R Archive Network.

Fig. 2.1), where you can download everything you'll need to use R (for free!). Having one site where everyone has to go to download all things R can result in some heavy network traffic, so there are actually mirror sites, or duplicates, of the CRAN website hosted at institutions all over the world. These sites are identical to the original CRAN site but allow for users to download the R software and R packages from networks much closer to home and with lower traffic. This can really speed up downloads and prevents the site from being swamped. Once you're on the CRAN main site, look for and click on the Mirrors link; it should be the top link of the left-hand menu. Find a country or institution that's close to you and click on the associated link. This will take you to a CRAN mirror site. Everything should look exactly the same, except you'll notice that the url is different. Now you can select one of the three links to download R for the operating system you're using. If you're using Windows you'll want to select Download R for Windows and then click the base link on the subsequent page to find the Download R #.#.# for Windows link. If you're using Mac OS you can select the Download R for (Mac) OS X link, then select the R-#.#.#.pkg link under the **Latest release:** label. If you are using an older distribution of Mac OS, there are instructions on this page on how to proceed depending on which version you are using. For Linux you can, hopefully unsurprisingly, select the Download R for Linux link to go to a list of directories. Each directory is specific to the distribution of Linux you are using, so if, for example, you were using Ubuntu, you would select the Ubuntu link and then look for the instructions under "To install the complete R system." Each of the download pages should have key information necessary for troubleshooting download and installation issues. If you run into difficulties, a web search describing either your error message or simply "installing R on" followed by the name of the operating system you're using should get you well on your way to troubleshooting most any issue that comes up.

If everything went well, you now have R installed on your computer. On Windows you can simply double click the R.exe icon (if you didn't make a desktop shortcut during installation, you should be able to find it in the bin folder in the larger R folder, by default located in Program Files). On Mac or Linux you can open up the command-line terminal and type in

```
R
```

Clicking the icon or typing in the above command should start up a command-line R session (Fig. 2.2). (Make sure it is a capital R, and if you

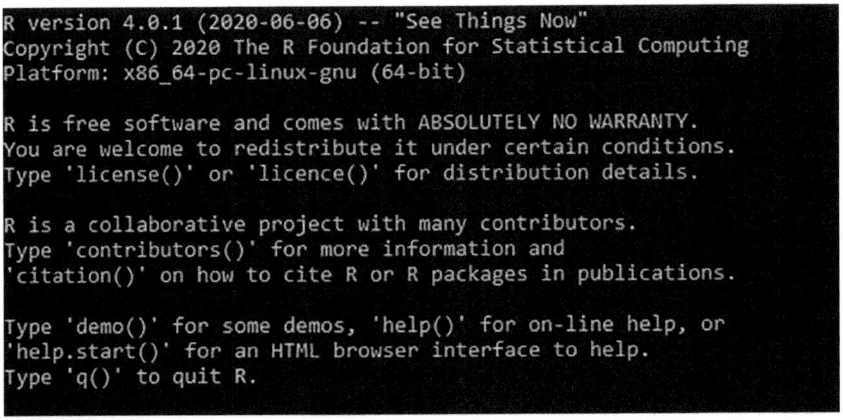

```
R version 4.0.1 (2020-06-06) -- "See Things Now"
Copyright (C) 2020 The R Foundation for Statistical Computing
Platform: x86_64-pc-linux-gnu (64-bit)

R is free software and comes with ABSOLUTELY NO WARRANTY.
You are welcome to redistribute it under certain conditions.
Type 'license()' or 'licence()' for distribution details.

R is a collaborative project with many contributors.
Type 'contributors()' for more information and
'citation()' on how to cite R or R packages in publications.

Type 'demo()' for some demos, 'help()' for on-line help, or
'help.start()' for an HTML browser interface to help.
Type 'q()' to quit R.
```

Figure 2.2 The basic R terminal screen.

get stuck in the session type `quit()` to get out.) Everything we cover in this book should function perfectly well from this command line. However, there have been some excellent GUIs developed for R that add some bells and whistles that can really help with keeping track of scripts, objects, help pages, and generated figures. A GUI is simply a system of graphics you can click on with a cursor to issue a command or make a selection, instead of typing it out on a terminal. A GUI we've used a lot is provided by RStudio, which, like R, is also free and easy to install. RStudio is technically an Integrated Development Environment (IDE) which comes with a GUI, but for now we're mostly interested in RStudio for GUI-related purposes. If you go to `http://www.rstudio.com`, you should be able to navigate to the option to download the RStudio Desktop installer for either a Windows, Mac, or Linux operating system (you have the option of purchasing a commercial license or downloading an RStudio server, but we will only be concerned with the free open-source licensed RStudio Desktop here). Once RStudio is successfully installed, you should open it up and see the four main areas of the GUI (Fig. 2.3).

The main terminal, the same terminal we saw in Fig. 2.2, should be visible in the bottom left pane. Directly above that, you effectively have a

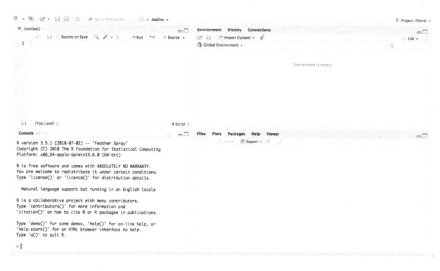

Figure 2.3 The RStudio main screen.

built-in text file that allows you to write in and edit your code before you execute it in the terminal. We'll be typing most of our code into that top-left window, then hitting the CTRL + ENTER or CMD + ENTER buttons on your keyboard, with the cursor next to our line of typed-out code to execute it in the terminal below. Right beside the terminal window, in the bottom right, there's another window that contains several tabs. The Files tab allows you to view the files on your computer and create new folders directly from within RStudio. The Plot tab is where figures you generate with your code will show up. The Packages tab shows you what R packages you've already installed on your computer as well as which ones you've already opened up in your current session (more on packages at the end of Chapter 9). The Help tab is where documentation files will pop up when you request more information on a function or package (we'll cover how to do that soon as well). Finally, the Viewer tab is where you can get RStudio to display files designed to be viewed as websites, such as HTML and Rmd files (we won't be getting into Rmd files in this book, but more advanced R users may want to familiarize themselves with the utility of R Markdown).

With RStudio now up and running, we can begin to play around a bit with some basic commands and execute a few simple tasks in R. The first thing we can attempt is to install the R package that's associated with this book, called *popgenr*. This is a very small package that mostly contains datasets we'd like you to have access to during certain exercises. To install this package, you can either type install.packages("popgenr") directly into the R terminal, or you can click on the Packages tab in RStudio and click on the Install button. This will open up a small search window where you can type in popgenr with no quotation marks, hit ENTER, and it should be installed with no problem. Note: you must be using at least R version 3.5 or later for the package to install and work properly.

2.2 Working directories and saving

To save R code that you've written in RStudio, simply press the floppy disk symbol above the text file window. R code can be written in any kind of basic text editor (it's generally not a good idea to write programming code in an editor that adds a lot of behind-the-scenes formatting, like Microsoft Word or Apple Pages, but rather use editors like Linux Xed, Microsoft Notepad, or Apple TextEdit, to give just three basic examples). If you want to specify that a text file contains R code—we'll call these files R scripts—the text at the end of the file name (the file extension) should be". R". All R code saved from RStudio will have this ". R" extension by default, but if you're using a basic text editor and not an R GUI, the file will probably default to being saved with the ".txt" file extension. This should be easy to change manually from your desktop by either clicking on the file name or right clicking and selecting Rename and replacing ".txt" with ". R". The benefit of having a dedicated file extension for your code is that you can keep better track of your files and set default methods of handling code files with a specified programming language extension. There are many script file extensions specific to individual programming languages such as ". R" for R scripts, ". py" for Python scripts, ". pl" for Perl scripts, and ". cpp" for C++ scripts, to name just a few. When saving anything from within R or RStudio, all files will be output to what's called your working directory. There's a default working directory that R defines whenever you open up a new R session. You can see what this default directory is by typing getwd() into the R terminal. This will look something like this:

```
> getwd()
[1] "/Users/yournamehere"
```

In order to change this working directory, you just have to run another very similar command on the R terminal setwd(). Let's say we want to change our working directory to a folder on our desktop called R_project. We can do that like so:

```
> setwd("/Users/yournamehere/Desktop/R_project")
```

Note that if you're on Windows, the directory location might be formatted a little differently. Unlike Mac or Linux operating systems, Windows uses backslashes "\," not "forward" slashes "/."

In RStudio you can also use the GUI to change working directories. At the very top of the RStudio window, simply select `Session`, then `Set Working Directory`, and finally `Choose Directory`. This will bring up a new window where you can use your cursor to select the folder you want to set as your working directory. Now we can start actually playing around with some inputs and calculations!

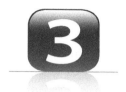

Basic Commands in R

⊣ Term Definitions ⊢

Functional Programming: A way to program based on applying methods consistently, regardless of the nature of the data.

Logical value: Also sometimes called Boolean values, they are the response to a logical expression such as "Is **x** greater than **y**?" In R the logical values are TRUE, FALSE, NA ("Not Available"), and NaN ("Not a Number").

Matrix: An array of numbers organized by rows and columns that can organize complex processes and undergo mathematical operations.

Multivariate: Something containing or considering multiple variables at once.

Object-Oriented Programming (OOP): A way to program based on grouping and classifying specific data as objects, then executing different methods on that object given its class.

Vector: A data structure that contains multiple elements of the same type.

3.1 Input and calculations

Now that we have R up and running, we can begin to play around with it a little bit. If you're using the base R installation, you can type code into the command-line window, and if you're using RStudio, you can input code in the bottom left window, the terminal (refer back to Chapter 2 if you're

Population Genetics with R: An Introduction for Life Scientists. Áki J. Láruson and Floyd A. Reed, Oxford University Press (2021). © Áki J. Láruson & Floyd A. Reed.
DOI: 10.1093/oso/9780198829539.003.0003

unclear on how to identify the terminal). To start with, you can use R as a large calculator. Using standard mathematical operators (+, −, *, /) you can type a few simple calculations directly into the R command line.

```
> 2+2
[1]  4

> 6-5
[1]  1

> 4*7
[1]  28

> 100/5
[1]  20
```

You can sometimes express operations in a couple of different ways. If you wanted to input 3 to the power of 2 (that is, 3^2), you could do this by inputting any of the following:

```
> 3*3
[1]  9

> 3^2
[1]  9

> 3**2
[1]  9
```

R follows a standard order of operations (in order of priority: exponents, multiplication or division, addition or subtraction), and parentheses can be used to modify the order. To verify, we can type in:

```
> 8/2^3+2*3
```

If R were to simply read in each input left to right and execute it, we'd end up with an output of 198. Instead, we see:

```
> 8/2^3+2*3
[1]  7
```

So R is first calculating the exponential term ($2^3 = 8$), then moving left to right calculating each multiplication or division in the order they were input, starting with $8/8 = 1$, then $2 * 3 = 6$. Finally, it adds the result of these calculations $(1 + 6)$ to end up with 7. If we wanted to force a strict left-to-right calculation, we could do so using parentheses:

```
> (((8/2)^3)+2)*3
[1]  198
```

These are all pretty short and sweet commands that we're inputting; however, as we start creating longer and slightly more complex codes we are going to want to move away from typing things directly into the command line and instead type out our commands in a text file that we can then execute on the command-line terminal. In RStudio, the top-left window provides just such a feature: you can type in and edit several lines of commands in this built-in editor, before selecting the section you want to execute and pressing CTRL + ENTER or CMD + ENTER to execute them. If you have your flashing text cursor (also called a "caret") on a specific line, executing will input that specific line into the command-line terminal. If you want more than one line, you'll have to highlight all that you want executed before issuing the command. If you want to execute everything written in the window, you can highlight everything with CTRL + A or CMD + A or simply press the Source button on the top right of that window. When a file containing code is "sourced," the entire code in the file is executed by R.

While we will continue to display commands as if they were being input directly into the command line, with a primary ">," we encourage you to start typing out commands in a generic text file or in the RStudio editor window. It's worth mentioning again, just like we did in Chapter 1, that there's no need to ever type in ">" at the beginning of your code. It is only there to signal the beginning of the command-line input, and is there automatically on your terminal.

3.2 Assigning objects to variables

R uses both object-oriented and functional programming paradigms (Chambers 2014). What that means is that R generally behaves like a calculator that computes consistently without regard for the type of data being input (functional), but also has the ability to consider specifically declared objects as having a preferred approach (object-oriented). This will hopefully become clearer once we introduce the different classes of objects, but for now let's simply jump into creating an object. An object is defined by having both data and a name, so to start let's create an object named x that consists of a series of numbers ranging from 1 to 10.

To get this vector of numbers we can actually do a few different things. We can combine each individual number using the combine function c():

```
> c(1,2,3,4,5,6,7,8,9,10)
[1]   1   2   3   4   5   6   7   8   9 10
```

or we can use the operator : to specify the range of numbers:

```
> 1:10
[1]   1   2   3   4   5   6   7   8   9 10
```

or we can use another function, seq(), to declare a sequence ranging from 1 to 10:

```
> seq(10)
[1]   1   2   3   4   5   6   7   8   9 10
```

Let's stick with seq() for now, and create our object. We want to name our object x, and we can do this like so:

```
> x <- seq(10)
```

We have now assigned our data (numbers 1 through 10) to a variable (x) and have created our first object. Congratulations! We could also have used the operator = instead of < - to assign the variable, but since = comes up in many different contexts we'll stick to assigning variables with < -. If we wanted to, we could even flip the order and assign x like this:

```
> seq(10)  -> x
```

While that's radical, in this book we'll be consistently placing our variables on the left.

You can check the value of x at any time within R by typing

```
> print(x)
[1]   1  2  3  4  5  6  7  8  9 10
```

Finally, one powerful aspect of vectors is that you can perform operations on the entire vector at once. Let's multiply x by three.

```
> x*3
[1]   3  6  9 12 15 18 21 24 27 30
```

3.3 Parts of a function

Notice that the function seq() can be run with only one argument: the final value of the sequence. By default, seq() starts at 1 and increases by 1 up until the final value is reached. Functions in R generally have some minimum number of arguments that need to be specified before they'll run, but they can also have many more options than just those minimally required. For example, seq() can take three different arguments at once. The function could be written like this: seq(from, to, by). When only one value is given to seq(), it'll assume that from and by are both equal to 1. So we could get the exact same output if we input:

```
> seq(1, 10, 1)
[1]   1   2   3   4   5   6   7   8   9  10
```

To find out exactly what arguments a function takes, you can look up a help file from directly within R. To look up the vignette associated with any distributed function in R, you can type in ?function() or help(function) and the R Documentation help file will pop up. If you're using the base R installation, the help file will open up either in your command line (you'll need to press "q" to close it) or in your default web browser, depending on your operating system. If you're using RStudio, the help file will pop up in the bottom-right window, under the Help tab, regardless of what operating system you're using. If you look up the help file for seq(), you'll see a general description of the function, followed by the set-up for general usage. In this usage section, you'll notice that the arguments seq() can take are actually named:

```
Usage

seq(...)

## Default S3 method:
seq(from = 1, to = 1, by = ((to - from)/(length.out - 1)),
  length.out = NULL, along.with = NULL, ...)
```

Notice the comment (demarcated by ##) that this is a "Default S3 method." R has three underlying object-oriented systems, or object models, that it uses to handle object classes. These systems are called S3, S4, and Reference Classes (RC). This function was designed to explicitly work with the S3 system. Don't worry too much about these distinctions until you start writing your own R packages.

In the above vignette you can also see that seq() has at least five named arguments: from, to, by, length.out, and along.with. Notice that from, to, and by all have values associated with them: a default value of 1 for both from and to, and a value for by based on from and `to`. The arguments `length.out` and `along.with` both have a default value of NULL. This implies that they have no default value and must be explicitly assigned a value in order to be utilized. Also notice that there is an order to the arguments in the function. By default, the function will interpret any argument values given to it in the order specified in the help file. This is how we're able to type in `seq(1, 10, 1)` and get the implied `from = 1, to = 10, by = 1` output. If we don't want to rely on the order and actually be explicit, we can assign the argument values by using their names. Doing this allows us to put the arguments in any order we want, as long as we've named them correctly:

```
> seq(to = 10, by = 1, from = 1)
[1]  1  2  3  4  5  6  7  8  9 10
```

If we don't want to go with the default of "starting from 1" and "increase by 1" we can assign different values to those arguments. Let's create another object, called y, and assign to it a sequence going from 2 to 20 by increments of 2. To get that, we'd simply put:

```
> y <-  seq(from = 2,  to = 20,  by = 2)
```

Now we do want to see the sequence of numbers we just made. So to view the contents of an object we can simply input the name of it in the command line:

```
> y
[1]  2  4  6  8 10 12 14 16 18 20
```

We should now have two objects already saved in our terminal. You can type in the function `ls()` to see what objects are currently saved in your environment:

```
>  ls()
[1] "x" "y"
```

If you're using RStudio, you'll also be able to see the objects you've saved in the upper right-hand window, under the `Environment` tab.

So we have two vectors of numbers saved in our environment. Let's combine these two vectors into a data frame with the use of the well-named function `data.frame()`:

```
>    data.frame(x,y)
       x   y
1      1   2
2      2   4
3      3   6
4      4   8
5      5  10
6      6  12
7      7  14
8      8  16
9      9  18
10    10  20
```

Our output here is a data frame with ten rows, each numbered by default and shown on the far left, and two columns by default named after their assigned variables x and y. One very important thing to note here is that the nice new data frame we just made has not been saved. It has been output following our command but does not exist as an object in our R environment. Let's actually save our data frame so we can start to manipulate it. We'll do this by assigning our data frame to some variable. Let's save our data frame as `datf`:

```
> datf <-   data.frame(x,y)
```

3.4 Classes of objects

So, we've now made several objects (remember, you can view all objects with the command `ls()` or a glance at the `Environment` tab in RStudio), and we've even generated objects with different classes! To see what class our objects are let's use the function `class()`:

```
>   ls()
[1]  "datf"  "x"  "y"

>   class(datf)
[1]  "data.frame"

>   class(x)
[1]  "integer"

>   class(y)
[1]  "numeric"
```

Our data frame datf appears to be a class called "data.frame"; a little on the nose, but let's be grateful for something so straightforward.
What doesn't seem immediately straightforward is that x and y have two
different classes! In R, objects of class "integer" and class "numeric" are
pretty similar; in fact, "integer" is a subset of "numeric" and is simply
a number that cannot take a decimal value. This distinction is made in
R mostly as a memory-saving strategy, since saving a discrete variable
(integer) takes less memory than saving a continuous variable (numeric).
But how did we end up with these two different classes for values that were
generated by the same function? The difference was in what arguments
we used in the function: when we assigned x we used seq(10), whereas
when we assigned y we used seq(from = 2, to = 20, by = 2).
The more explicit way of calling the function seq() allows for the option
to end up with decimals, say if we specified that we wanted a range from 0 to
1 in 0.1 increments, while the more simplistic way with only one argument
specified can only produce integers. It's important to be aware of the classes
of objects you're making, because certain functions may only be able to
handle certain classes and not others.

Let's try making another object, this time using a constant that's been
built into R, called letters. This constant contains all twenty-six letters
of the modern English alphabet in their lower-case forms. You can also call
all the letters in their upper-case forms with LETTERS:

```
> letters
 [1] "a" "b" "c" "d" "e" "f" "g" "h" "i" "j" "k" "l" "m"
[14] "n" "o" "p" "q" "r" "s" "t" "u" "v" "w" "x" "y" "z"

> LETTERS
 [1] "A" "B" "C" "D" "E" "F" "G" "H" "I" "J" "K" "L" "M"
[14] "N" "O" "P" "Q" "R" "S" "T" "U" "V" "W" "X" "Y" "Z"
```

Notice that the output above extends outside the normal width of the command line and therefore continues on the next line, starting with the number of the first output element on the new line (that is, "n" is the fourteenth letter of the alphabet and therefore the fourteenth component of the output).

But we don't necessarily want all twenty-six letters in our object. Let's say we only want the first ten; in this case, we can do what's called "subsetting," where we take a subset from a set of data. One way to do this is to place brackets after the object and express a numeric range within them. Let's save this new subset as variable z:

```
> z <- letters[1:10]
```

Usually when we assign a variable, R doesn't output whatever you just put in there. So, if you want to view what was actually saved as you assign it, you can place the whole expression within parentheses and then R will call the variable once everything's assigned to it:

```
> (z <- letters[1:10])
 [1] "a" "b" "c" "d" "e" "f" "g" "h" "i" "j"
```

Let's now take a look at what class of object we've just made:

```
>  class(z)
[1] "character"
```

An object containing characters in programming is often called a "string." So we've now got an object that's a string (a vector of letters), which is of a class called "character," that's assigned to variable z. Our vocabulary is growing by leaps and bounds.

One of the main strengths of the class "data frame" is that it can take multiple classes of objects and keep track of these classes while remaining a "data frame." Let's make a data frame that contains both our numeric and string objects.

```
> (datf <-  data.frame(x,y,z))
      x  y z
1     1  2 a
2     2  4 b
3     3  6 c
4     4  8 d
5     5 10 e
6     6 12 f
7     7 14 g
8     8 16 h
9     9 18 i
10   10 20 j
```

We can see what this new object contains, but let's take a closer look at what it's actually made of. There are two functions which can quickly give us a summary and the structure of our objects. Those functions are summary() and str(), which stands for "structure."

Let's see what these functions can tell us about our new objects.

```
>  summary(datf)
        x              y           z
 Min.   : 1.00   Min.   : 2.0   a      :1
 1st Qu.: 3.25   1st Qu.: 6.5   b      :1
 Median : 5.50   Median :11.0   c      :1
 Mean   : 5.50   Mean   :11.0   d      :1
 3rd Qu.: 7.75   3rd Qu.:15.5   e      :1
 Max.   :10.00   Max.   :20.0   f      :1
                                (Other):4

>  str(datf)
```

```
$ x: int   1 2 3 4 5 6 7 8 9 10
$ y: num   2 4 6 8 10 12 14 16 18 20
$ z: Factor w/ 10 levels "a","b","c","d",..: 1 2 3 4 5 6 7
8 9 10
```

We see that `summary()` gives us a numeric breakdown of columns x and y, with a six-number summary (Minimum, First Quartile, Median, Mean, Third Quartile, and Maximum) for both. For z we see a tabulation of the number of occurrences of each element within z. The reason for these differences is that the objects that make up `datf` have different classes, but `summary()` doesn't say anything explicitly about the different classes at play here. Meanwhile, `str()` gives us explicitly which class each object belongs to right from the start, labeling x as class `int` (for "Integer"), y as class num (for "Numeric"), and z as a `Factor`.[1] A breakdown of what elements are contained in each object follows this class distinction. For x and y, this consists simply of the elements they contain. For z, we see `Factor w/ 10 levels "a"`, a `"b"`,...etc. But hold on—we already looked at the class of z earlier and it was of the class "character." So why is `str()` telling us a different class? Let's try using the function `class()` again, but specifically on z within the `datf` object. We can isolate any individual column within a data frame by appending the name of the column after the name of the data frame, separated by the symbol "$."

```
> datf$x
 [1]  1  2  3  4  5  6  7  8  9 10

> datf$y
 [1]  2  4  6  8 10 12 14 16 18 20

> datf$z
[1] a b c d e f g h i j
Levels: a b c d e f g h i j
```

Now that we know how to isolate individual columns in a data frame, we can easily apply functions to these specific subsets of our data. So now look

---

[1] If you're using R version 4.0+ characters are not automatically converted to factors in data frames.

at the `class()` of column z and compare it with the class of stand-alone object z:

```
>   class(datf$z)
[1]  "factor"

>   class(z)
[1]  "character"
```

The class of column z is definitely different from the class of object z; how can that be? Well, part of the object-oriented nature of R is that sometimes it will redefine classes of variables as they're linked to other variables. In this case, R redefined our "character" string to a "factor." Note that this exact scenario will not take place if you're using the most recent distribution of R, but it's worth referencing here since its important to keep track of the object classes within data frames. What a "factor" does is take a series of inputs and make each element its own category. So now, instead of having a string of letters, we have a set of ten categories, named "a" through "j." This can be quite useful, as you'll hopefully see later, but it can also become the source of confusion when suddenly a certain function won't run correctly because an object's class was changed without your explicit command to do so. Functions `class()`, `summary()`, and `str()` are excellent components of your tool box when it comes to spot checking and troubleshooting code.

3.5 Matrices

You should now have a pretty good sense of how to assign objects to variables, find the classes of objects, combine different objects into data frames, and subset individual columns of these data frames. Data frames are very useful formats for storing and manipulating data, especially data containing multiple classes. But there's another way to store data that we want to cover before we continue, and that is as a matrix. Unlike data frames, matrices in R only take elements of the same class. So you can't have a single matrix of both numbers and factors, only one or the other.

The benefit of this is that mathematically manipulating matrices is often a lot more straightforward than with data frames. Let's start by making our first matrix, containing the elements from x and y. Begin by looking up the help file for the function matrix(). Notice that matrix() can take five arguments: data, nrow, ncol, byrow, and dimnames. We want the data in our matrix to consist of the values contained in x and y, so in order to input that data through a single argument we'll need to use the combine function c() that we used earlier:

```
>  c(x,y)
[1]   1   2   3   4   5   6   7   8   9  10   2   4   6   8  10  12  14
[18]  16  18  20
```

Obviously we don't want our matrix to be a jumble of numbers, but with this single vector of numbers we'll seed our matrix. We specifically want all the elements from x (the first ten variables in the combined jumble above) to be in the first column of our matrix, then all the elements from y (the subsequent ten elements in the jumble) to make up the second column. We'll specify this using the nrow and ncol arguments by setting the number of rows (nrow) equal to 10 and the number of columns (ncol) equal to 2. Now let's make this matrix, which we can name Neo:

```
>  (Neo <- matrix(data = c(x,y),   nrow=10,   ncol=2))
          [,1] [,2]
 [1,]      1    2
 [2,]      2    4
 [3,]      3    6
 [4,]      4    8
 [5,]      5   10
 [6,]      6   12
 [7,]      7   14
 [8,]      8   16
 [9,]      9   18
[10,]     10   20
```

Voilà! Our first matrix is up and running. Notice that each element of the data we specified for the matrix was seeded by filling in the ten-element long column first, before moving into the second column. This order of seeding the matrix was specified by the argument `byrow`, which is by default set to the logical value FALSE. If we change that FALSE to TRUE we'll see something a little different.

```
> matrix( data = c(x,y),   nrow = 10,   ncol = 2,   byrow = TRUE
         [,1]  [,2]
 [1,]     1     2
 [2,]     3     4
 [3,]     5     6
 [4,]     7     8
 [5,]     9    10
 [6,]     2     4
 [7,]     6     8
 [8,]    10    12
 [9,]    14    16
[10,]    18    20
```

You'll notice that the columns are now a mixture of elements from both x and y, since the matrix was seeded by filling in elements across the two columns before moving down to the next row.

One thing to mention here is that R does pay attention to capital letters. If you attempt to call the matrix without the capitalization, R will have no idea what you mean:

```
> neo
Error: object 'neo' not found
```

Now that we have our matrix, we can begin to manipulate it in a distinct way which will be important later in this book: by using matrix multiplication. If you're not already familiar with matrix multiplication, we'll give a very brief description here. Matrix multiplication is a remarkable way to consider multivariate changes. When you multiply two matrices together, you're not just considering the individual effects of two numbers on each other, but also their positions relative to other elements within the matrix. Because of these positional effects, the way matrices are multiplied takes into consideration both row and column elements. Multiplying a matrix by a single number is easy enough. Let's see what happens when we multiply our matrix, Neo, by 2.

```
> 2 * Neo
       [,1]  [,2]
 [1,]    2     4
 [2,]    4     8
 [3,]    6    12
 [4,]    8    16
 [5,]   10    20
 [6,]   12    24
 [7,]   14    28
 [8,]   16    32
 [9,]   18    36
[10,]   20    40
```

Each element of the matrix is simply multiplied by the single numerical value. But now let's consider two matrices being multiplied together. Let's start by making a small matrix, a, such that

$$a = \begin{bmatrix} 1 & 2 \\ 3 & 4 \end{bmatrix}.$$

We can make a by seeding a two-row by two-column matrix with a vector containing the numbers 1 through 4, making sure to first fill in all elements in each row before moving on to the next row.

```
> (a <- matrix(c(1:4), nrow=2, ncol=2, byrow=TRUE))
       [,1]  [,2]
 [1,]    1     2
 [2,]    3     4
```

Let's think of a matrix A that has i number of rows and j number of columns (an i x j matrix) and a matrix B which is a j x k matrix. The way matrix multiplication progresses is by summing the products of each element in each of the i rows in matrix A and each of the columns k in matrix B, so you end up with an i x k matrix. This can be expressed like so:

$$\begin{bmatrix} A_{1,1} & A_{1,2} \\ A_{2,1} & A_{2,2} \end{bmatrix} X \begin{bmatrix} B_{1,1} & B_{1,2} \\ B_{2,1} & B_{2,2} \end{bmatrix} = \begin{bmatrix} \sum_{j=1}^{2} (A_{1,j} * B_{j,1}) & \sum_{j=1}^{2} (A_{1,j} * B_{j,2}) \\ \sum_{j=1}^{2} (A_{2,j} * B_{j,1}) & \sum_{j=1}^{2} (A_{2,j} * B_{j,2}) \end{bmatrix}$$

You may notice that when we talk about an i x j matrix and a j x k matrix, there's a shared term, j, between them. This is because while you can readily multiply matrices with differing i and k dimensions, you cannot use this approach to multiply matrices that don't share a j term. Which is to say that the number of columns in the first matrix must be the same as the number of rows in the second matrix.

If we multiply the matrix a that we just made by itself, we can calculate the resulting matrix using the same approach:

$$\begin{bmatrix} 1 & 2 \\ 3 & 4 \end{bmatrix} X \begin{bmatrix} 1 & 2 \\ 3 & 4 \end{bmatrix} = \begin{bmatrix} (1 * 1) + (2 * 3) & (1 * 2) + (2 * 4) \\ (3 * 1) + (4 * 3) & (3 * 2) + (4 * 4) \end{bmatrix} = \begin{bmatrix} 7 & 10 \\ 15 & 22 \end{bmatrix}$$

So let's see what happens when we multiply a by itself in R

```
> a * a
        [,1] [,2]
[1,]     1    4
[2,]     9   16
```

What is that?! It appears that each value was simply multiplied by itself, regardless of its row or column placement. *This is not matrix multiplication.* What's happened here is that R multiplied two sets of numbers, with no regard for the matrix class to which those numbers belong. In R you need to explicitly specify matrix multiplication by replacing the "*" with a "%*%." Let's see what we get when we specify matrix multiplication

```
> a %*% a
        [,1] [,2]
```

```
[1,]     7    10
[2,]    15    22
```

That looks more like it. Alright, so we can multiply square matrices pretty readily, but now let's make two matrices with differing numbers of dimensions called b and c that each have five elements (in this case the numbers 1 through 5), but let's make b have 5 rows and 1 column and c have 1 row and 5 columns.

```
> (b <- matrix(c(1:5), nrow=5, ncol=1))
       [,1]
[1,]     1
[2,]     2
[3,]     3
[4,]     4
[5,]     5

> (c <- matrix(c(1:5),nrow=1, ncol=5))
       [,1] [,2] [,3] [,4] [,5]
[1,]     1    2    3    4    5
```

Notice how c is effectively the same matrix as b, but flipped around so it has the opposite number of rows/columns. This arrangement can be called the transpose of b. There's already an R function that can give you the transpose of any matrix, so we could have created the exact same matrix c using function t():

```
> (c <- t(b))
       [,1] [,2] [,3] [,4] [,5]
[1,]     1    2    3    4    5
```

Now that we have these two matrices with different dimensions, let's see what happens when we again try to multiply these matrices with just the "*" command.

```
> b * c
Error in b * c : non-conformable arrays
```

Because "*" doesn't automatically consider the matrix approach, if the dimensions of the matrices are different it can't simply multiply each corresponding element in either matrix. So now let's properly multiply our 5×1 and 1×5 matrices; this should progress exactly the same way as with a above, except since there are 5 rows in the first matrix (corresponding to i above) and 5 columns in the second matrix (k) we expect the calculation to progress like so:

$$
\begin{bmatrix}
\sum_{j=1}^{1}(A_{1,j}*B_{j,1}) & \sum_{j=1}^{1}(A_{1,j}*B_{j,2}) & \sum_{j=1}^{1}(A_{1,j}*B_{j,3}) & \sum_{j=1}^{1}(A_{1,j}*B_{j,4}) & \sum_{j=1}^{1}(A_{1,j}*B_{j,5}) \\
\sum_{j=1}^{1}(A_{2,j}*B_{j,1}) & \sum_{j=1}^{1}(A_{2,j}*B_{j,2}) & \sum_{j=1}^{1}(A_{2,j}*B_{j,3}) & \sum_{j=1}^{1}(A_{2,j}*B_{j,4}) & \sum_{j=1}^{1}(A_{2,j}*B_{j,5}) \\
\sum_{j=1}^{1}(A_{3,j}*B_{j,1}) & \sum_{j=1}^{1}(A_{3,j}*B_{j,2}) & \sum_{j=1}^{1}(A_{3,j}*B_{j,3}) & \sum_{j=1}^{1}(A_{3,j}*B_{j,4}) & \sum_{j=1}^{1}(A_{3,j}*B_{j,5}) \\
\sum_{j=1}^{1}(A_{4,j}*B_{j,1}) & \sum_{j=1}^{1}(A_{4,j}*B_{j,2}) & \sum_{j=1}^{1}(A_{4,j}*B_{j,3}) & \sum_{j=1}^{1}(A_{4,j}*B_{j,4}) & \sum_{j=1}^{1}(A_{4,j}*B_{j,5}) \\
\sum_{j=1}^{1}(A_{5,j}*B_{j,1}) & \sum_{j=1}^{1}(A_{5,j}*B_{j,2}) & \sum_{j=1}^{1}(A_{5,j}*B_{j,3}) & \sum_{j=1}^{1}(A_{5,j}*B_{j,4}) & \sum_{j=1}^{1}(A_{5,j}*B_{j,5})
\end{bmatrix}
$$

This shows us that we should see a 5×5 matrix as a result of this matrix multiplication. Let's see what we actually get.

```
> b %*% c
      [,1] [,2] [,3] [,4] [,5]
[1,]    1    2    3    4    5
[2,]    2    4    6    8   10
[3,]    3    6    9   12   15
[4,]    4    8   12   16   20
[5,]    5   10   15   20   25
```

Let's just make sure that everything is behaving as we expect. We can spot check the row 5 column 5 element in the matrix based on our above equations:

$$
\sum_{j=1}^{1}(b_{5,j}*c_{j,5}) =
$$

$$
(b_{5,1}*c_{1,5}) = (5*5) = 25
$$

Alright, that seems to pan out. But now what if we flip the order in which we multiply these matrices? Instead of our 5×1 multiplied by our 1×5, we multiply our 1×5 by 5×1. What dimensions do you expect the resulting matrix to have? Let's try it out and see what we get.

```
> c %*% b
         [,1]
[1,]     55
```

This should make sense if we think about the formula

$$\sum_{j=1}^{5} (c_{1,j} * b_{j,1}) =$$

$$(c_{1,1} * b_{1,1}) + (c_{1,2} * b_{2,1}) + (c_{1,3} * b_{3,1}) + (c_{1,4} * b_{4,1}) + (c_{1,5} * b_{5,1}) =$$

$$(1 * 1) + (2 * 2) + (3 * 3) + (4 * 4) + (5 * 5) =$$

$$1 + 4 + 9 + 16 + 25 = 55.$$

So this should make it clear that the order by which you multiply matrices makes a pretty big difference.

Now that we have the tools to assign variables, manipulate data frames, generate matrices, and execute matrix multiplication, we should be well equipped to employ some basic population genetics probability calculations in R.

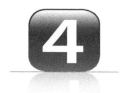

Allele and Genotype Frequencies

⊢ Term Definitions ⊢

Allele: A genetic variant.

Diploid: An individual with two copies of all (most) genetic material.

Haploid: An individual with one copy of all genetic material.

Heterozygote: An individual with differing copies of an allele.

Homozygote: An individual with identical copies of an allele.

Genotype: The combination of alleles in an individual.

Locus: Physical location of an allele, plural *loci*.

Phenotype: The physical result of a genotype (and nongenetic influences).

4.1 Introduction to population genetics

Much of population genetics concerns itself with establishing expectations for genetic variants, or alleles, in a population. How many individuals are expected to be carrying a certain allele? How probable is it to find two copies of a rare mutation? How likely is a certain genotype to be from one population or another? If we have an underlying expectation for how these alleles should behave under very simple assumptions, we can start to

Population Genetics with R: An Introduction for Life Scientists. Áki J. Láruson and Floyd A. Reed,
Oxford University Press (2021). © Áki J. Láruson & Floyd A. Reed.
DOI: 10.1093/oso/9780198829539.003.0004

look for deviations from these expectations to make insightful predictions regarding population dynamics. Let's start with some very rudimentary expectations of frequency and probability.

We will be very general in our definition of an "allele." In classical genetics, an allele can be defined as a variant of a gene that leads to a different phenotype, either as a heterozygote or homozygote. Here we are using the term allele to mean any genetic variant (mutation) at a specific locus or position within a genome, regardless of its effect (if any) on genes or phenotypes. A very common type of mutation is a single nucleotide variation, also called a Single Nucleotide Polymorphism or SNP. For example, if a copy of the DNA sequence ... GTAG[C]TAGAC... were to change to ...GTAG[T]TAGAC..., we would see that the C nucleotide highlighted by the brackets in the first sequence had changed to a T. If we compared multiple copies of this DNA sequence, we would see that the site, or locus, inside the brackets is a polymorphic locus, since there are two alleles associated with it (C or T). We'll focus a lot on diploid examples in this book, since organisms that have two copies of their genome in every cell are pretty common and include such interesting creatures as Peacock Spiders (*Maratus volans*), Brown Algae (*Ascophyllum nodosum*), and Humans (*Homo sapiens*). And since we're assuming diploidy, we know that having two alleles at a single locus means that we can have three different possible genotypes: CC, CT, and TT.

This hypothetical T allele will be at some frequency, p, in a population. This fraction p can be at any value from zero to one. If we randomly draw an allele from this population, then the probability of picking the T allele is equal to its frequency p. If the frequency of an allele is 1/2 in a population, then the probability of an individual inheriting one copy of the allele from one parent is also 1/2 (in the absence of any additional information about the genotype of the parent). So half the individuals in a new generation are expected to inherit the T allele from one of their parents *and* some of those individuals will also inherit a T allele from their other parent, again with a probability of 1/2. Half of half of all individuals in the new generation will then be expected to have two T copies. The frequency of these homozygotes is expected to be $p \times p = p^2$. Implicit here is the assumption that these variants are effectively randomly inherited. We'll have to make a lot of assumptions when modeling something as complex as the genetics of populations over time, but we'll cover those assumptions in more detail later.

For now, we can calculate the above example within an R session by setting the allele frequency as object p:

```
> p <- 0.5
```

Then the frequency of homozygotes is $1/2 \times 1/2 = 1/4$:

```
> p^2
[1] 0.25
```

This uses the multiplication rule of probability for independent events. We're assuming that the chance of inheriting a T allele from your mother is *independent* of the probability of inheriting the same allele from your father; thus, we can multiply the probabilities together.

We can also work backward from an observed genotype frequency to an expected allele frequency. Some genetic variants result in recessive phenotypes when they are homozygous. Say we observe homozygotes with a new mutant allele at a frequency of one out of 1,000 in a population:

```
> f <- 1/1000
```

Since this is the frequency of p^2 (homozygotes), we can take the square root of this to estimate the allele frequency p with the function sqrt(),

```
> sqrt(f)
[1] 0.03162278
```

which is approximately three out of 100 (≈ 0.0316). What is the expected frequency of carriers (heterozygotes) that only have one copy of the mutant allele? If the probability of inheriting an allele is p, then probability of *not* inheriting it is $1 - p$ (there are only two outcomes here, and the total of all possible outcomes has to sum to 100%). This is the subtraction rule of probability. Because we are only interested here in the heterozygous case, these individuals *either* inherited one copy of the allele from their mother but not their father, $p(1 - p)$, *or* did not inherit a copy from their mother but did from their father, also $(1 - p)p$. These two events are mutually exclusive: the mutant allele came either from the mother *or* the father in order for the individual to be a carrier. So, we use the "or" (additive) rule of probability and add the different outcomes together: $p(1-p)+(1-p)p = 2p(1 - p)$.

These expectations of a p^2 homozygote frequency and a $2p(1 - p)$ heterozygote frequency are known as the Hardy–Weinberg genotype proportions.

Box 4.1

The Hardy–Weinberg principle is a bedrock of classical population genetics. This principle is centered around the mathematical expectation for the interplay of allele and genotype frequencies. It is essentially a binomial expansion of $(p + q)^2$ to $p^2 + 2pq+q^2$, where q stands in for $1-p$. This is an example of a scientific idea whose "time had come," in that multiple parties independently came to very similar conclusions all around the same time. However, the principle is usually only named after two of these parties: the mathematician Godfrey H. Hardy from England and the physician Wilhelm Weinberg from Germany. They both published papers in 1908 detailing the expectations we've just gone through here (Edwards 2008). Hardy's paper ("Mendelian Proportions in a Mixed Population") was a letter to the editor of *Science*. It focused on correcting a misconception regarding how prevalent a condition known as brachydactyly, characterized by short fingers and toes, is expected to be over multiple generations. Weinberg's paper ("*Über den Nachweis der Vererbung beim Menschen*," which translates to "On the Proof of Heredity in Humans") focused generally on the expectations of genetic inheritance in a randomly mating population. The Hardy–Weinberg principle allows us to make solid predictions of genotype proportions, and although there are a number of assumptions inherent in this principle, as we'll see later in this chapter, it holds up remarkably well in real-world situations.

To continue with our example, if an allele exists in a population at some frequency p, then homozygotes are expected to occur at a frequency of p^2 and heterozygotes at a frequency of $2p(1 - p)$ in that population. We can observe these expected genotype frequencies over a range of possible allele frequencies by plotting this relationship.

Let's use a built-in function called curve(). If you just enter curve without the parentheses into your R terminal you'll see the full code that defines the function. This can be a useful feature. In R you can always look under the hood, so to speak, of most any function you're using by typing in only the name of said function.

Try opening the help file for curve() now. From the help file you should be able to see that the curve() function requires, first and foremost, some expression to plot. Since we're interested in plotting homozygote frequencies (which can be expressed as p^2) over a range of allele frequencies from zero to one, we can start by typing in:

```
> curve(x^2, 0, 1)
```

You should see a generated image with a nice smooth line representing the relation between x on the x-axis and x^2 on the y-axis between zero and one, similar to the plot in Fig. 4.1.

Note that we're using the variable x in the command instead of p. This is simply because x is quite often the default stand-in variable in the R language. The function will not run if you replace x with another character. Now let's get a bit more fancy. Plot this relationship again, but this time

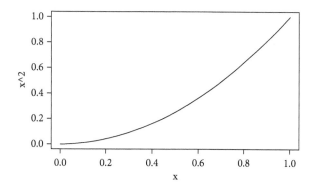

Figure 4.1 Output of the function "curve" plotting x^2 against x.

specify what our x- and y-axes represent. We can do this by adding in the xlab (x label) and ylab arguments. Also, give this line a specific color via the col argument and make the line a little bit thicker with the lwd (line width) argument. Our input is now

```
> curve(x^2, 0, 1, xlab = "Allele frequencies",
    ylab = "Genotype frequencies", col = "green", lwd = 2)
```

Remember from Chapter 3 that it doesn't matter in what order you place your arguments (col before xlab, for example) as long as you've specified their names inside the function. We've now plotted the expected relationship between increasing frequencies of a specific allele and homozygous genotype frequencies. Next let's add a label to this curve. For that we'll use the aptly named function text() which will, perhaps not surprisingly, add text to our plot. We'll have to give the text() function x- and y-coordinates on which to place our text, and let's make our text the same color as our line by using the col argument again:

```
> text(0.6, 0.2, "Homozygotes", col = "green")
```

We now have a green label centered at x = 0.6 and y = 0.2 that identifies our expected homozygous genotype frequencies. You should see a figure similar to Fig. 4.2.

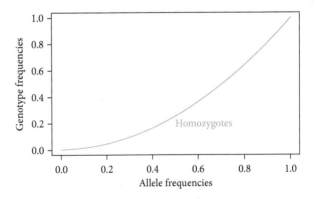

Figure 4.2 Relationship of allele frequency, p, to expected homozygote genotype frequency, p^2.

What can we infer from this plotted relationship? The plot shows that as the frequency of a certain variant (allele) increases, the frequency of diploid individuals carrying two copies of this variant also increases. This should make intuitive sense: as an allele becomes more common in a population the probability that both parents pass this allele on to their offspring increases.

Now let's add the expected heterozygote genotype frequencies to this plot. Remember that heterozygote frequencies are expected to follow $2p(1-p)$, so let's again use the "curve" function, but this time plotting $2*x*(1-x)$ instead of x^2, and let's make this line blue. Also, in order for this curve to show up on the same plot we already made for our homozygote expectation, instead of starting over with a new plot we need to include the argument add = TRUE.

```
> curve(2*x*(1-x), 0, 1, add=TRUE, xlab="Allele frequencies",
    ylab="Genotype frequencies", col="blue", lwd=2)

> text(0.25, 0.5, "Heterozygotes", col = "blue")
```

All that together should give the following plot (Fig. 4.3).

Here we're seeing different frequency expectations for heterozygotes and homozygotes as the allele frequency increases. Tracking the increase from left to right across the x-axis, as the allele increases in frequency there is at first a more rapid increase in the number of heterozygotes than in the number of homozygotes. But as you approach the 50% allele frequency the number of heterozygotes levels off, and once you have a sizable majority (well over 50%) of the population carrying this allele more individuals start carrying two copies of it as homozygotes than are carrying only one copy of it as heterozygotes. When an allele frequency reaches 1.0 (100%), the allele is said to have become "fixed" in the population. Once that happens it can only exist in homozygous individuals, because there are no other variant alleles around. When an allele frequency reaches 0.0 (0%), that allele is said to be "lost" or "extinct."

There is clearly a point on the plot where for some allele frequency you expect an equal number of homozygotes and heterozygotes. Let's find this

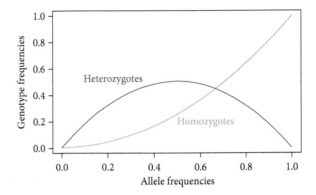

Figure 4.3 Expected homozygote and heterozygote genotype frequencies as a function of allele frequencies. Note that when an allele is rare (with an allele frequency of much less than 0.5) it exists in the population mostly in heterozygotes. When it is more common (with an allele frequency of much greater than 0.5) it is more often found in homozygotes.

point and highlight it on the plot. First let's set the two equations equal to each other:

$$p^2 = 2p(1 - p).$$

Then expand the heterozygote estimate to get

$$p^2 = 2p - 2p^2.$$

Simplify this to

$$p = 2 - 2p,$$

which then gives us

$$p = 2/3.$$

When the value of p is equal to 2/3, the equation $p^2 = 2p(1-p)$ should be true. R is able to assess logical operators such as less-than ($<$), greater-than ($>$), and equal to ($==$). For example,

```
> 2+2 == 4
```

returns the value TRUE, whereas

```
> 2+2 == 5
[1] FALSE
```

Just to reiterate what we've mentioned before regarding assigning variables, evaluating whether two values are equal (p $==$ 1/2) is different from setting one variable equal to a value with a single equal sign (p $=$ 1/2). This is why some R programmers (like us) want to avoid confusion and always use $<$ - instead of $=$ to assign variables.

So, we should be able to check that the equation $p^2 = 2p(1 - p)$ is true when $p = 2/3$ quite easily by setting "p" to this value:

```
> p <- 2/3
```

and then seeing what we get when we input

```
> p^2 == 2*p*(1-p)
```

Surprisingly, this returns a FALSE.

This is the result of a rounding error that arises because of the way R (like many other languages and programs) saves long decimals. We can get around this by using the function all.equal(), which can logically assess "near equality" when that is a concern. When we input

```
> all.equal(p^2 , 2*p*(1-p))
```

we should get a validating TRUE.

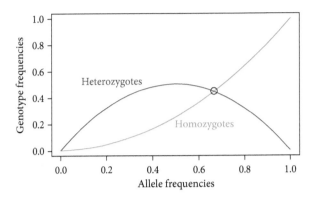

Figure 4.4 Highlighting the intersection of the heterozygous and homozygous genotype expectations.

Now, with the previous plot still open, we can edit it by adding points and lines as we like. Let's add a point where we expect the genotype frequencies of heterozygotes and homozygotes to be equal. For this, we'll use yet another aptly named function: `points()`. We'll need to specify an x-coordinate (2/3, or we can just input our previous variable p, since we have already set it equal to 2/3) and a y-coordinate (which can be p^2, $2p(1 - p)$, or simply $(2/3)^2$). Just like before with the curves we'll use `lwd` to thicken the outline of the point, but we're also going to expand the point slightly with the `cex` (character expansion) argument so that it's not just a small dot.

```
> points(p,p^2,lwd=2,cex=2)
```

We should now see a circle right at the point where the two curves intersect (Fig. 4.4).

Finally, we can save the code we've written so far in a text file so that we don't have to input it all again. All together, this is how our input should look:

```
> curve(x^2, 0, 1, xlab="Allele frequencies",
  ylab="Genotype frequencies", col="green", lwd=2)
```

```
> text(0.6, 0.2, "Homozygotes", col="green")

> curve(2*x*(1-x), 0, 1, add=TRUE, xlab="Allele frequencies",
    ylab="Genotype frequencies", col="blue", lwd=2)

> text(0.25, 0.5, "Heterozygotes", col = "blue")

> p <- 2/3

> points(p, p^2, lwd=2, cex=2)
```

Once again, remember that it is unnecessary to save the > in the written code. They are just visual place holders for each new input line of code.

Expected allele and genotype frequencies are just the beginning of population genetics. As we will see later, alleles can deviate from these expected proportions; however, in a range of cases these predictions are very robust. Hardy–Weinberg proportions are a population genetics null model of the absence of evolution. The forces that can cause evolutionary change (genetic drift, migration, mutation, selection, and recombination) will be visited in later chapters.

At this point we have some working code that we've written out. It would be a good idea to save this code as a file that we can come back to later (or in case we mess it all up and need to re-load what we did earlier). Let's save this code as an R script called HW1.R (remember from Chapter 2 that the .R at the end defines this file as R code). Remember to make sure the R script is in your working directory (which you can change with setwd(); again, refer back to Chapter 2 for clarification) and then you can execute the whole script from within an R session with

```
> source("HW1.R")
```

This will execute all the code written in the script, so use the source command with caution if you're not interested in generating all the output of a script in one go.

4.2 Simulating genotypes

Often it helps guide our intuition of a process if we can simulate it and see how the simulations match, or do not match, what we expect. Let's simulate Hardy–Weinberg genotype proportions. First we're going to make a list of alleles to choose from to make up a population:

```
> allele <- c("A","A","a","a","a","a","a","a","a","a")
```

The variable `allele` is a vector of two *A* allele copies and eight *a* allele copies, which gives an *A* allele frequency of 2/10 or 20%. Instead of typing out a series of "A"s and "a"s, we can actually use a handy R function called `rep()`. This function lets us type a character or number we want to repeat and then simply say how often we want it repeated:

```
> allele <- c(rep("A",2), rep("a",8))
```

Notice how we combine the output of the two `rep()` functions with a `c()` function. These two ways produce the exact same object:

```
> print(allele)
 [1] "A" "A" "a" "a" "a" "a" "a" "a" "a" "a"
```

Next we create a matrix to record the alleles of individuals in the population. We start with a variable `popsize`, initially set to 100, which we can easily change later to model different population sizes.

```
> popsize <- 100
```

We then use the `matrix()` function to create a matrix of 100 rows (defined by `nrow = popsize`) and two columns (`ncol = 2`, because we're obsessed with diploids) and save it as pop.

```
> pop <- matrix(nrow=popsize, ncol=2)
```

Each row will correspond to an individual and the two columns represent the two copies of each locus where we'll be recording the alleles of that individual.

Now we are going to randomly choose alleles to make up our individual genotypes using R's built-in `sample` function. We're also going to employ what's called a loop, specifically a `for` loop. A `for` loop specifies how many times some set of tasks is to be performed. It essentially says "do this `for` this many iterations."

```
> for(i in 1:popsize){
    pop[i,1] <- sample(allele,1)
    pop[i,2] <- sample(allele,1)
}
```

This `for` loop moves from one all the way up to the `popsize` number, and uses a variable `i` to keep track of the current position. In the `pop` matrix individual `i` is assigned an allele. `sample(allele,1)` means copy one random entry out of the `allele` vector and `pop[i,#]` means record it in the corresponding position (row `i`, column `#`) in the matrix. Let's see what we've got after running this loop.

```
> pop
      [,1] [,2]
[1,]  "a"  "A"
[2,]  "a"  "a"
[3,]  "a"  "a"
[4,]  "a"  "a"
[5,]  "a"  "a"
[6,]  "a"  "a"
[7,]  "a"  "a"
[8,]  "a"  "A"
[9,]  "a"  "a"
[10,] "A"  "A"
[11,] "a"  "a"
[12,] "a"  "a"
 . . .
```

So, in this example, individual one is an a/A heterozygote and individual two is an a/a homozygote. (Each time this is run the result will be different because of the random sampling.) Notice that row numbers are represented first in the brackets and columns second ([row, column]). One way to subset data in R is by using brackets following a dataset name; specifying numbers within the brackets can pinpoint specific row and column coordinates.

Now we'll work through this matrix and calculate the A allele frequency, which will differ slightly between runs because of the random sampling of alleles. First we define a variable used to count the number of As that are found and initially set it to zero.

```
> Account <- 0
```

Then we need to go through the matrix and simply increase the count by one each time we see an A allele. For each individual we need to look at both the first and second positions. We'll be using conditional if statements to assess which allele is present. if statements are set up in a similar way to for loops, (function(condition){command}), but if statements are special in that they only progress to the command if the output from the condition is TRUE. The position in the matrix is designated by x and y within brackets following the matrix object: pop[x,y].

```
> for(i in 1:popsize){
    if(pop[i,1]=="A"){
        Account <- Account+1
    }
    if(pop[i,2]=="A"){
        Account <- Account+1
    }
}
```

The above code is going through each individual and asking if the allele stored in the first or second position is equal to A (if(pop[i,"1 or 2"]=="A")); if so, one is added to the current Account total.

Next we divide the count of A alleles by the total number of allele copies present in the population (`popsize` × 2 because each individual has two alleles) and save this A frequency as `AFreq`.

```
> AFreq <- Acount/(popsize*2)
```

This should give a value near 0.2. The actual value will vary a bit from 20% because of variation in the number of each allele sampled when R generates the dataset.

Now we will calculate genotype frequencies by going through the matrix again and counting how often heterozygotes appear, which can happen in two ways (A/a and a/A), and how often A/A homozygotes appear. Right now we're only focusing on the A allele, but later, once we know the heterozygote and A/A homozygote frequencies, we can calculate the remaining a/a homozygotes by subtracting from the total. We're going to add a new statement into the mix now: we're going to use `else`, which is only activated if the condition in the `if` statement is not met.

```
> Hcount <- 0

> AAcount <- 0

> for(i in 1:popsize){
    if(pop[i,1]=="A"){
        if(pop[i,2]=="a"){
            Hcount <- Hcount+1
        }else{
            AAcount <- AAcount+1
        }
    }
    if(pop[i,1]=="a"){
        if(pop[i,2]=="A"){
            Hcount <- Hcount+1
        }
    }
}
```

Just to quickly break down what we've done here: We create two counting variables, Hcount and AAcount, to keep track of our number of heterozygotes and our AA homozygotes, respectively. Then we loop through all the rows in pop, and if the first column contains an A, we check to see if the second column contains an a. If it does, we increase our heterozygosity counter by one. If it doesn't, we know it must be an A and our `else` statement is activated, increasing our AA homozygosity counter by one. If our first column instead contains an a, we check if our second column contains an A, and if so, increase our heterozygosity counter, because we don't mind if the heterozygote has an Aa or aA genotype.

Now that we have the number of heterozygotes and the number of A/A homozygotes, we can finally convert these genotype counts into frequencies:

```
> HetFreq <- Hcount/(popsize)

> AAFreq <- AAcount/(popsize)
```

Notice that we don't need to multiply popsize by two here because we're not dealing with individual alleles anymore, but genotypes corresponding to individuals. We can look at all the frequency variables we've saved so far with `print`:

```
> print(c(AFreq, HetFreq, AAFreq))
[1] 0.24 0.36 0.06
```

Now let's plot these simulated frequencies along with the p^2, $2p(1-p)$, and $(1-p)^2$ predictions for all three genotypes (A/A, A/a, and a/a). The following commands will plot the points using the `plot()` function. `par(new = TRUE)` is used to keep each preceding plot so multiple points can be added.

```
> plot(AFreq, HetFreq, xlab="allele frequency", ylab=" ",
    ylim=c(0, 1), xlim=c(0, 1), col="blue")

> par(new=TRUE)
```

```
> plot (AFreq, AAFreq, xlab=" ", ylab=" ",
  ylim=c(0, 1), xlim=c(0, 1), col="green")

> par(new=TRUE)

> plot (AFreq, 1-AAFreq-HetFreq, xlab=" ",
    ylab="genotype frequency", ylim=c(0, 1), xlim=c(0, 1),
    col="red")
```

Notice that the last point, the frequency of a/a homozygotes, is one minus the frequency of A/A homozygotes and A/a heterozygotes. This is because once you've accounted for two genotype frequencies in a bi-allelic system (two alleles at a locus; for example, A and a) the last genotype frequency constitutes the remainder, since there are only three possible genotypes (for example AA, Aa, aa). We wrapped the plot () function lines to an indented new line to keep the code to a readable width.

Finally, we add the predictions of the expected genotype frequencies with curve (), and labels are added with text () as in the last section.

```
> curve (2*x*(1-x), 0, 1, add=TRUE, ylab=NULL, lwd=2,
    ylim=c(0, 1), col="darkblue")

> curve (x**2, 0, 1, add=TRUE, ylab=NULL, lwd=2,
    ylim=c(0, 1), col="darkgreen")

> curve ((1-x)**2, 0, 1, add=TRUE, ylab=NULL, lwd=2,
    ylim=c(0, 1), col="darkred")

> text (0.5, 0.7, "Aa", col = "blue")

> text (0.9, 0.7, "AA", col = "green")

> text (0.1, 0.7, "aa", col = "red")
```

The result should look similar to Fig. 4.5. Note there are additional details such as the options set in the plot () and curve () functions

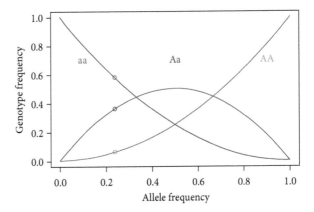

Figure 4.5 Plot of a simulation of sampling alleles into three genotypes (circles) and comparing to Hardy–Weinberg predictions (curves).

(for example, `xlab`, `ylim`, `lwd`, etc.) that were used to set up the plotting parameters. We've seen these options before so we're not going into the details of each of these, but don't be thrown by all the "window dressing" options. Also don't be afraid to change these values to see what happens and look up more details and options on your own.

Okay, that works fine for plotting a single point, but we are often interested in the distribution of many points. Let's change the code to run through some replicates and plot them simultaneously. Every time we run the simulation we'll draw a new allele frequency, so the greater the number of replicates we run, the greater the range of allele frequencies we'll see. To do this we will define the allele and genotype frequency as numeric vectors to record the different values by adding this code near the beginning of the script:

```
> AFreq <- numeric()

> HetFreq <- numeric()

> AAFreq <- numeric()
```

Then we'll create a new variable for the number of replicates to run and set up a loop that surrounds both the sampling steps and the calculation of frequencies (within the outside set of braces {...}). The modified center of code of the script looks like this:

```
> replicates <- 10 #Run ten simulations
> for(j in 1:replicates){ #Beginning of the replicate loop
    for(i in 1:popsize){ #Randomly sample alleles
        pop[i,1] <- sample(allele,1)
        pop[i,2] <- sample(allele,1)
    } #Close of the allele sampling loop
    Acount <- 0 #Count of A alleles
    for(i in 1:popsize){
        if(pop[i,1]=="A"){
            Acount <- Acount+1
            }
        if(pop[i,2]=="A"){
            Acount <- Acount+1
            }
    } #Close of the A allele count loop
    AFreq[j] <- Acount/(popsize*2) #Calculate A freq.
    Hcount <- 0 #Count of heterozygotes
    AAcount <- 0 #Count of AA homozygotes
    for(i in 1:popsize){ #Count genotypes
        if(pop[i,1]=="A"){
            if(pop[i,2]=="a"){
                Hcount <- Hcount+1
            }else{
                AAcount <- AAcount+1
            }
        }
    if(pop[i,1]=="a"){
        if(pop[i,2]=="A"){
            Hcount <- Hcount+1
            }
        }
    } #Close the genotype countin loop
    HetFreq[j] <- Hcount/(popsize) #Calculate het. freq.
    AAFreq[j] <- AAcount/(popsize) #Calculate hom. freq.
} #Close of the replicate loop
```

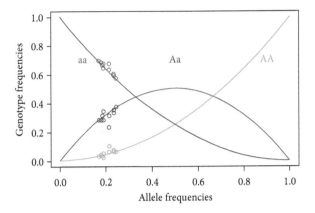

Figure 4.6 Plot of ten replicate simulations of sampling alleles into three genotypes (circles) and comparing to Hardy–Weinberg predictions (curves).

The number of the replicates is kept track of with a variable j. The printing of values to the command line within the replicate loop has been removed. Afreq, HetFreq, and AAFreq have been modified to keep multiple values and store each new value at position j in their lists: Afreq[j], HetFreq[j], and AAFreq[j]. Also notice that everything within the replicate loop has been indented to make the code easier to visualize. This is not necessary to do in R, but can be helpful when reading through your code. Running the full modified code, along with the plotting code on pages 50–51, gives a result similar to Fig. 4.6.

Up to this point, these simulations have been run by sampling allele frequencies centered on $p = 0.2$ from the original "allele" list (two "A"s out of the ten total). However, we can change the code to run across the entire range of possible allele frequencies.

At the beginning of the replicates loop, so directly following 'for(j in 1:replicates) {', we can add the simple command

```
p <- runif(1)
```

This sets p equal to a single random number drawn from a uniform distribution between zero and one (runif() stands for "random uniform," not "run if"). We can modify the set-up for the pop matrix so that the allele is randomly determined based on this p allele frequency by using a random draw, instead of the original sample(allele,1) assignment for pop[i,1] and pop[i,2]. We'll determine whether the allele is "A" or "a" by setting every runif() draw under the p threshold as an "A" allele and every draw over the threshold as an "a" allele. So, in our code from earlier, replace

```
for(i in 1:popsize){ #Randomly sample alleles
    pop[i,1] <- sample(allele,1)
    pop[i,2] <- sample(allele,1)
}
```

with

```
for(i in 1:popsize){
    if(runif(1)<p){
        pop[i,1] <- "A"
    }else{
        pop[i,1] <- "a"
    }
    if(runif(1)<p){
        pop[i,2] <- "A"
    }else{
        pop[i,2] <- "a"
    }
}
```

Let's run 1,000 replicates (by specifying replicates <- 1000) and see what we get. After this runs, you should be seeing something similar to Fig. 4.7.

This begins to illustrate the power of using programs to simulate processes. One thousand outcomes were generated and plotted much faster than we could ever do by hand. In general, the simulation matches the prediction. However, details such as the larger variance in heterozygotes

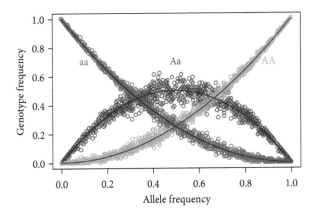

Figure 4.7 Plot of 1,000 replicate simulations of sampling alleles into three genotypes (circles) and comparing to Hardy–Weinberg predictions (curves) over the entire possible range of allele frequencies.

around $p = 1/2$ become apparent. Try running the code with different population sizes and numbers of replicates. What would you expect to see in a population of ten individuals versus a population of 100?

4.3 Calculating allele frequencies from datasets

We've now gone through made up and simulated data to get a feel for the quite logical theory behind how alleles behave in a population, but do these models of expected genotype frequencies work in the real world? How close are these predictions to the frequencies in reality?

If we have the genotypes of individuals in a population sample, then we don't have to assume Hardy-Weinberg proportions to estimate the allele frequency from phenotype frequencies. We can simply count the alleles. Each heterozygote has one copy of the allele and a homozygote has two copies (again assuming a diploid organism). Since each individual sampled has two copies of each locus, the total number of alleles observed is twice the number of individuals sampled.

We can then calculate the frequency of a specific allele by adding the number of heterozygotes to two times the number of homozygotes (since each homozygote has two copies of the allele) and divide that by two times the number of individuals sampled (since each sampled individual carries two loci):

$$p = \frac{2m + t}{2n}$$

Here above, m is the number of homozygotes, t is the number of heterozygotes, and n is the total number of sampled individuals. We can simplify this to

$$p = \frac{m + t/2}{n}.$$

Box 4.2 - Hardy–Weinberg assumptions

We've mentioned several times the assumptions underlying our Hardy–Weinberg expectations. But what exactly are all of these assumptions? In order to get to $p^2 + 2pq + q^2$ and run the simulation we used here to illustrate expectations, the following assumptions are made:

- The organisms being considered are diploid.
- The organisms being considered are exclusively reproducing sexually (no cloning).
- There are not distinct populations present with different allele frequencies, with or without migration among them.
- The population we're considering is effectively infinite in size.
- All mating occurs randomly.
- No genetic variant is being affected by natural selection (differences in survival and reproduction of the alleles).
- No genetic variants are lost or gained because of mutation (no allele mutates into a new allele).
- Generations don't overlap. Once reproduction occurs, all the parents disappear and only the resulting offspring contribute to the subsequent generation.

Obviously these expectations are not very biologically realistic. However, Hardy–Weinberg expectations are surprisingly robust to violations in most of these assumptions, except for the first three: haploid or polyploid organisms have to be treated in a different, but logical, way, organisms reproducing asexually can deviate greatly from Hardy–Weinberg expectations, and population subdivisions can cause significant deviations.

Table 4.1 Observed number of carriers (Het.) and affected individuals (Hom.) for three recessive disease phenotypes: cystic fibrosis (CF), sickle cell anemia (SC), and β-thalassemia (βT). Data adapted from Lazarin et al. 2013.

Disease	n	Het.	Hom.
CF	23,369	842	9
SC	21,360	307	2
βT	21,096	158	1

Now let's look at some real-world genotype data. In Table 4.1, we see the results of an international screen of tens of thousands of individuals for three potentially disease-causing alleles, and whether the person screened was homozygous or heterozygous for the allele.

Let's start by looking at the number of individuals from the screening that are homozygous for cystic fibrosis (CF): this number (9) suggests that there are eighteen total CF alleles being carried by these nine individuals. Now the number of carriers (heterozygotes) is quite a bit larger (842), which we might expect to be the case for a rare allele (refer back to Fig. 4.3). Let's calculate the allele frequency for the CF allele using $p = \dfrac{m + t/2}{n}$:

```
> p <- (9+842/2)/23369
```

Be sure to use the parentheses here as they preserve our order of operations.

From our above calculation we should now have a variable p with a value of 0.01840045, so an allele frequency of about 1.8%. If you'd like to see the results of your calculation displayed, even while saving it as a variable, you can put the whole input in parentheses like so:

```
> (p <- (9+842/2)/23369)
[1] 0.01840045
```

This will output the result as well as save the variable.

Now we have an allele frequency value (an estimate of the population frequency from a sample) that's been calculated directly from observed data. Under the assumptions of the Hardy–Weinberg principle, we expect that we can calculate the number of heterozygotes from this allele frequency with the formula $2p(1-p)$. Thus our expected frequency of carriers can be calculated as

```
> 2*p*(1-p)
 [1] 0.03612374
```

which gives us an expected heterozygote genotype frequency of about 3.6%. How does this compare to the real observation of the heterozygote genotype frequency? A total of 842 heterozygotes were observed out of the 23,369 people screened. That's 842/23,369, which is equal to $\approx$0.03603, or about 3.6%. The difference between what's expected and what's observed is remarkably small. Let's perform the same calculation for sickle cell anemia (SC) and β-thalassemia (βT). Compiling these values into Table 4.2, we see that $2p(1-p)$ is a remarkably good predictor of the observed frequency of heterozygotes.

Incidentally, we can also see that the frequency of carriers (heterozygotes) is much higher than the frequency of affected individuals (homozygotes) for recessive genetic disorders. This follows Hardy–Weinberg predictions (again, refer back to Fig. 4.3). The ratio of heterozygotes to homozygotes is predicted to be

$$\frac{2p(1-p)}{p^2} = \frac{2(1-p)}{p} \approx \frac{2}{p},$$

Table 4.2 Comparing expectations of Het. frequency [$2p(1-p)$] to the actual observed frequency.

Disease	p	Het. expected	Het. observed
CF	0.0184	0.036124	0.036031
SC	0.00728	0.014454	0.014373
βT	0.00380	0.007556	0.007490

with the implication that when an allele is rare (that is, p is very small), $1-p$ is approximately equal to 1. Try

```
> curve(2/x, 1e-7, 0.01, log="y")
```

to visualize this relationship on a log scale.

For a more general correspondence between Hardy–Weinberg predictions and actual observations let's take a look at a larger dataset. If you were able to successfully install our *popgenr* package (refer back to Chapter 2 for instructions), we can now make use of it. Before accessing anything from installed packages, they have to be loaded with the command `library()`.

```
> library("popgenr")
```

Now, having loaded the R package *popgenr*, you can load a bundled dataset called `snp` by entering the command

```
> data(snp)
```

which contains twenty-five haphazardly sampled allele and genotype frequencies from across the human genome and should now be loaded as object `snp`. This `snp` dataset is a subset from the 1,000 Genomes Project (`http://www.internationalgenome.org`), a public repository of known human genetic variants from across the globe. There are a few different ways in which a dataset like this can be saved in R, and we specifically need to know the "class" of this dataset before we are able to properly work with it:

```
> class(snp)
[1] "data.frame"
```

Now that we know that we have an object of class `data.frame`, let's take a look at what we've just loaded. We could just type in the object name to see the whole thing, but if working with large datasets, or if we just want to spot check that everything looks alright, we can use the command `head()` to look at the first six lines of a dataset, like so:

```
> head(snp)
          ID      p     hom    het chromosome        type
1   rs200000  0.364  0.145  0.439          5  intergenic
2   rs300000  0.281  0.080  0.403         16  intergenic
3   rs500000  0.381  0.157  0.448          8    upstream
4   rs600000  0.023  0.002  0.042         22    upstream
5   rs700000  0.055  0.005  0.099          6      intron
6  rs1000000  0.166  0.027  0.278         12    upstream
```

If we want to see more rows than the default six, we can modify the
head() command by adding an integer after the dataset name, separated
by a comma (for example, head(dataset, 10)). We can see that this
dataset is a table with column names: ID, which is the unique Reference
SNP cluster ID for that variant; p, which is the allele frequency for that
SNP; hom and het, which are the homozygous and heterozygous genotype
frequencies, respectively; chromosome, which names the chromosome in
the human genome where that SNP is located; finally, we have a column
called type. This column contains more specific information about the
location of the SNP, but we'll look at that more later. First let's look at the
element types within this data frame by using the command str():

```
> str(snp)
'data.frame' :    25 obs. of  6 variables:
 $ ID         : Factor w/ 25 levels "rs1000000","rs1100000",...
 $ p          : num   0.364 0.281 0.381 0.023 0.055 0.166 0.406
 $ hom        : num   0.145 0.08 0.157 0.002 0.005 0.027 0.167
 $ het        : num   0.439 0.403 0.448 0.042 0.099 0.278 0.478
 $ chromosome : int   5 16 8 22 6 12 21 13 14 16 . . .
 $ type       : Factor w/ 7 levels "3UTR","downstream", . . .
```

You can refer back to Chapter 3 for more details on classes in R and the
output from str(). From the output above, we can see that we have
25 observations (rows) of 6 variables (columns) and that there are three
different types of elements in this dataset. $ID and $type are both listed
as factors. One nice thing about "factor" classes is that they are quite handy
when you want to summarize across categories. For example, if you enter

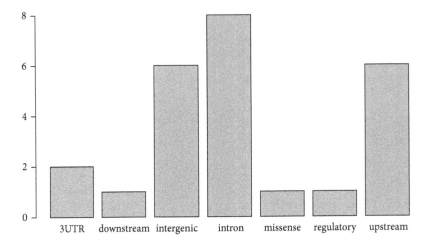

Figure 4.8 A barplot of the different locations of the SNPs in our dataset, relative to coding genes.

```
> plot(snp$type)
```

R will give you a barplot of the number of observations in each "type" category (Fig. 4.8). Notice that most of these SNPs are located in introns, followed by intergenic and upstream regions. These terms are defined and visualized in Box 4.3. The columns $p, $hom, and $het are all type numeric (num), while column $chromosome contains integers (int).

Now that we have a feel for the layout of our dataset, let's plot the allele and genotype frequencies from the snp data frame as points on the previous plot that we made (Fig. 4.3). The allele frequency of each variant in the file is stored in the $p column, while the homozygous and heterozygous genotype frequencies are stored in $hom and $het, respectively. As a reminder, we generated Fig. 4.3 with the following code:

```
> curve(x^2, 0, 1, xlab="Allele frequencies",
    ylab="Genotype frequencies", col="green", lwd=2)
> text(0.6, 0.2, "Homozygotes", col="green")
> curve(2*x*(1-x), 0, 1, add=TRUE, xlab="Allele frequencies",
    ylab="Genotype frequencies", col="blue", lwd=2)
> text(0.25, 0.5, "Heterozygotes", col = "blue")
```

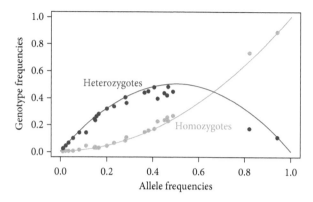

Figure 4.9 A plot of theoretical predictions of expected genotype frequencies (curves) and actual data (points) of human variation.

Now let's add in the allele ($p) and genotype frequencies ($hom & $het) from our snp dataset as points on our plot. Let's again use the points() function, but let's make the points a solid color by giving the pch (plotting character) argument a value of 19:

```
> points(snp$p, snp$hom, pch = 19, col = "green")
> points(snp$p, snp$het, pch = 19, col = "blue")
```

We should now have something similar to Fig. 4.9.

Overall there appears to be good agreement between the predictions and measured data. Several features are apparent. Deviations from the prediction are generally in a direction of less heterozygosity and more homozygosity than expected. This is consistent with demographic effects such as differences in allele frequency among populations, which will be discussed in more detail later. Also, notice that most of the points in the plot are at allele frequencies of less than 50%; this is because the variants we are plotting are a result of mutations creating new allelic variants (a derived state) from a pre-existing genetic sequence (an ancestral state determined by comparing to the closest relatives to humans), which would tend to start out being pretty rare. We'll revisit this idea again when we begin making predictions about random fluctuations in allele frequencies and discuss the concept of genetic drift.

Box 4.3 - SNP locations and types*

Upstream: The area before the gene sequence.
Intron: A space inside a gene sequence that is not included in the final product.
Missense: A SNP that changes the final product of the gene.
3'UTR: The UnTranslated Region at the end of a gene.
Intergenic: The area between two genes.
Regulatory: A sequence that regulates the expression of a gene.
Downstream: The area after the gene sequence.

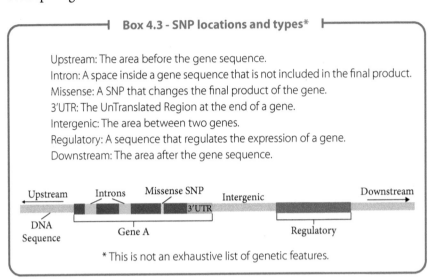

* This is not an exhaustive list of genetic features.

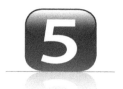

Statistical Tests and Algorithms

Term Definitions

Algorithm: A series of operations executed in a specific order.

Probability: The chance of an occurrence given repeated attempts.

Likelihood: The chance of an occurrence given a model assumption.

Machine Learning: A process where computational results are validated to improve accuracy.

Parthenogenesis: Development of an embryo without fertilization.

Autogamic: Self-fertilizing.

5.1 Deviation from expectations

At this point we've spent a fair amount of time validating that our expectations for allele frequencies under Hardy–Weinberg assumptions are reasonable. Now that we have a set of expectations that we believe, we have a powerful tool that we can use to compare and describe populations. One of the most interesting observations we can make is that a population is defying our expectations, and when that happens we can start to explore alternatives. One specific statistical tool we can use' in this exploration is called the χ^2 (chi-square; chi is pronounced kai) statistical test. We can use this test to see if our observed genotype frequencies are actually diverging from our expectations based on Hardy–Weinberg predictions.

Population Genetics with R: An Introduction for Life Scientists. Áki J. Láruson and Floyd A. Reed, Oxford University Press (2021). © Áki J. Láruson & Floyd A. Reed.
DOI: 10.1093/oso/9780198829539.003.0005

Let's look at a real dataset of genotype counts from samples donated by 501 people in Lagos, Nigeria (Taiwo et al. 2011). These are genotypes of a hemoglobin-producing gene which has the locus associated with sickle-cell anemia (hemoglobin S). First let's calculate allele and expected genotype frequencies, and then we can perform a χ^2 test on these data.

Begin by saving each of the observed genotype counts as their own variable. We'll use AA to denote homozygote non-sickle-cell genotypes, SS for homozygote sickle-cell allele genotypes, and AS for the heterozygotes:

```
> AA <- 366
> AS <- 123
> SS <- 12
```

The sum of these three genotype counts will give us the total number (n) of individuals:

```
> n <- AA+AS+SS
> print(paste("n:", n))
```

It is often useful to print a label to output along with our numeric results. This can help us keep track when there are multiple outputs from our code. Here we combined "n" with the number stored in n using the paste() function within the print() function. This returns

```
[1] "n: 501"
```

on the command line.

Now let's calculate the allele frequency of the S allele from the number of observed genotypes:

```
> p <- (SS + (AS/2))/n
> print(paste("p:", p))
[1] "p: 0.146706586826347"
```

Note that the parentheses around AS/2 are not necessary because R uses an appropriate order of operations, but we've added them to make sure it's clear that we're adding half the number of heterozygotes to the total number of homozygotes. With this observed allele frequency p we can now calculate our expected genotypes. Because we want to keep track of two different alleles (S & A) and therefore two different homozygosities, we'll define the SS homozygote as p^2 and the AA homozygote as $(1 - p)^2$. The implication here is that there are only two alleles possible: S at a frequency of p and A at a frequency of everything that is not p.

Now by multiplying our calculated genotype frequencies by the number of actual individuals sampled we can get the number of individual genotypes we expect:

```
> EAA <- n*(1-p)^2
> EAS <- n*2*p*(1-p)
> ESS <- n*p^2

> print(paste("Expected:", EAA, EAS, ESS))
[1] "Expected: 364.782934... 125.434131... 10.782934..."
```

To determine whether the number of genotypes we're seeing actually matches our expectations, we'll use a built-in R function, `pchisq()`, to calculate the probability value (*P*-value) from a χ^2 distribution. In the `pchisq()` function, we'll want to set the argument `lower.tail` to `FALSE`, because we want to see the probability of our χ^2 value being higher than it is. As our observations and expectations differ more and more our χ^2 value should increase, and loosely speaking the probability of getting a very large χ^2 value should get smaller and smaller. Let's start now by calculating a value for the χ^2 test statistic,

$$\chi^2 = \sum \frac{(E - O)^2}{E},$$

where E is the expected number of counts and O is the observed number of counts, and this is summed over all categories. We'll want to find where this χ^2 statistic falls in the distribution, but in order to have an appropriate distribution we'll have to tell the function how many degrees of freedom (df) to consider for the test. In general, we start with the number of categories of the data minus one when calculating degrees of freedom, so in this case three categories (EAA, EAS, and ESS) minus one. However, we also had to estimate a parameter from the observed data, p, to generate the expected values in each category. This means we've lost an additional degree of freedom. So, df $= 3 - 2 = 1$ (the expected numbers "fit" the observed data more closely by estimating a parameter from the observed data, so this comes at a cost):

```
> chi2 <- (EAA-AA)^2/EAA+
    (EAS-AS)^2/EAS+
    (ESS-SS)^2/ESS

> print(paste("chi-square:", chi2))

> pvalue <- pchisq(chi2, df = 1, lower.tail = FALSE)

> print(paste("P-value:", pvalue))
```

This code gives

```
[1] "chi-square 0.188666341317465"
[1] "P-value 0.664028935603698"
```

The resulting *P*-value is large (0.664), which suggests that our observed values are pretty much in line with our expected values (a common, but arbitrary, threshold is to say a value is significantly different from expectations if the *P*-value is less than 0.05 and, as in this case, we can ignore multiple testing issues). So this observed data appears to be entirely consistent with what we expected from Hardy–Weinberg predictions.

The χ^2 test is actually a convenient approximation of a likelihood ratio test known as the G-test, or the goodness-of-fit test, that is also commonly used to assess the correspondence between a model's predictions and actual real-world data:

$$G = 2\sum(O \times \log_e(O/E)).$$

This approach, as the name suggests, concerns itself with the ratio of the likelihoods of our observed values to the expected values. This G-test approach uses the same distribution as the χ^2 test and should perform similarly. The χ^2 test has usually been taught instead of the G-test because it doesn't require you to calculate log values; however, with the advent of electronic calculators (or computers in general), there's less need to shy away from more complex calculations, so let's also use this likelihood ratio approach to test our genotype observations. To try something different, let's set this up by manipulating vectors with multiple elements instead of individual objects like we did for the χ^2 test. We'll start by creating two vectors from our observed and expected numbers of genotypes, which will allow us to perform a slightly more streamlined calculation of the G-test statistic:

```
> geno <- c(AA, AS, SS)

> expe <- c(EAA, EAS, ESS)

> G <- 2 * sum(geno * log(geno/expe))

> print(paste("G:",G))
[1] "G: 0.184075382936793"

> pvalue <- pchisq(G, df = 1, lower.tail = FALSE)

> print(paste("P-value:", pvalue))
[1] "P-value: 0.667894063332523"
```

The resulting P-value (0.668) from this G-test is, as expected, very similar to the χ^2 test (0.664), so again we're pretty sure our observed data is not too different from our expectations. Note that for the G-test we have the same number of degrees of freedom, and lower.tail is again set to FALSE.

If you remember from Box 4.2 in the previous chapter, one of the conditions necessary for Hardy–Weinberg predictions is that no genetic variant is being affected by natural selection. Here we are working with alleles that have a significant effect on a phenotype, such as causing sickle cell anemia when homozygous and conferring resistance to malaria when heterozygous, and are clearly in violation of this assumption (Luzzatto 2012). But, as we saw from the hemoglobin S data we just analyzed, these assumptions can often be violated and yet the departure from Hardy–Weinberg expectations can appear quite small. Let's look at an example where this is not the case.

One of the Hardy–Weinberg assumptions is the effectively random union of gametes in each generation, regardless of the underlying allele frequency. This is strongly broken in clonal species, where a single parent produces an offspring that is genetically identical to itself. The water flea *Daphnia pulex* is one such species, where females typically reproduce by parthenogenesis (an unfertilized egg develops into an embryo) and some populations are even obligately parthenogenic (Paland et al. 2005; Fig. 5.1).

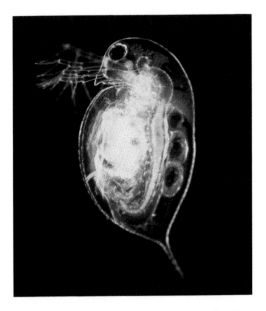

Figure 5.1 The water flea *Daphnia pulex*. So much research has focused on this species that it was the first crustacean to have its whole genome sequenced. Photo by Paul Hebert.

Let's look at an example of 118 individual *D. pulex* sampled from Charing Cross (the community in Ontario, Canada, not the London train station) who were genotyped for two alleles of phosphoglucose isomerase (PGI), which we'll again call "A" and "S" so we can reuse our previous code (Hebert and Crease 1983). One hundred AS heterozygotes and thirty-four AA homozygotes were found, while SS homozygotes were completely missing from the sample.

We can substitute these counts into the R script already written:

```
> AA <- 34
> AS <- 100
> SS <- 0

> n <- AA+AS+SS

> p <- (SS + (AS/2))/n

> EAA <- n*(1-p)^2
> EAS <- n*2*p*(1-p)
> ESS <- n*p^2

> geno <- c(AA,AS,SS)
> expe <- c(EAA,EAS,ESS)

> chi2 <- sum((expe-geno)^2/expe)

> print(paste("chi-square:",chi2))
[1] "chi-square: 47.4773242630385"

> pvalue <- pchisq(chi2, df=1, lower.tail=FALSE)

> print(paste("P-value:",pvalue))
[1] "P-value: 5.56438965556751e-12"
```

We can see that this is a significant departure from our expectation, with a *P*-value of 5.56×10^{-12}, and we can conclude that at least one of these variants in the PGI gene may have something more going on than is to be expected under Hardy–Weinberg conditions; that is, that we do not have random union of gametes in each new generation.

We can visualize these data as a barplot using the R function `barplot()`. We do need to set up our data a little specifically so that the `barplot()` function reads it in correctly, so we'll start by creating a matrix of our data (that we'll creatively call `dat`) where our two vectors each make up a row. You can always revisit Chapter 3 for a refresher on the `matrix()` function:

```
> dat <- matrix(c(geno,expe), nrow = 2, byrow = T)
```

Next we'll call the `barplot` function, specify that we want our two rows to be plotted `beside` each other, flag some interesting colors with the `col` argument, and finally add labels with `names.arg`:

```
> barplot(dat,beside=T,
    col=c("turquoise4", "sienna1"),
    names.arg=c("AA", "SA", "SS"))
```

One last step we want to take, is add a legend to this barplot which tells us what the two nifty colors we specified represent. To do that, we just run the `legend` command once we've generated our initial figure to specify that our two `legend` values, `Observed` and `Expected`, correspond to the two color (`col`) values `turquoise4` and `sienna1`. For placement, we can specify the keyword `topright` instead of giving an x-coordinate:

```
> legend(x="topright", legend=c("Observed","Expected"),
    pch=15, col=c("turquoise4","sienna1"))
```

Now we can look at our barplot and hopefully be pretty convinced that the sample is significantly different from what we'd expect under Hardy–Weinberg assumptions (Fig. 5.2).

In these examples we're dealing with relatively small numbers, and ideally the χ^2 test depends on the assumption that large samples have been

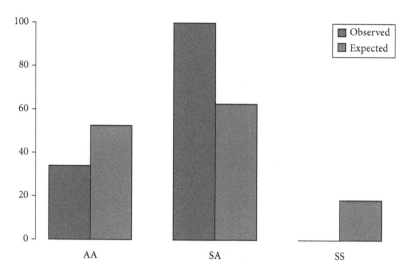

Figure 5.2 Barplot of observed versus expected genotype numbers in the PGI gene.

taken. Alternative methods of testing are considered more appropriate in situations where you're dealing with smaller sample sizes, such as an "exact test" where all possible genotype configurations of the alleles are used to assign a *P*-value to the observed configuration. See Guo and Thompson (1992), Wigginton et al. (2005), Engels (2009), and references therein for further discussion of exact tests in this context. However, in general, these different statistical approaches will be consistent with each other in terms of final interpretation if sample sizes are sufficient to test the size of the effect of interest and results near the boundaries of significance cut-offs are not focused on too seriously (for example, Johnson 1999).

5.2 Extending to more than two alleles

So far we've been focusing on a two-allele (bi-allelic) system where the allele frequency of one allele is expressed as *p* and the allele frequency of the other is expressed as $(1 - p)$. However, genotype predictions can easily be extended to more than two alleles. Since we're always assuming fully random mating, our theoretically expected number of homozygotes is still

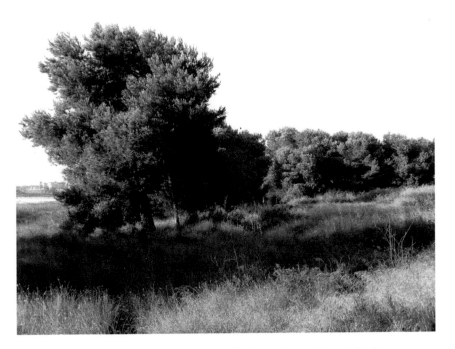

Figure 5.3 A grove of Aleppo pine, *Pinus halepensis*, near Torrevieja, Spain. Photo by Javier Martin.

going to be based on p^2 for each allele, regardless of how many alleles we're considering. The expected homozygosity of a set of j alleles is therefore the sum of the squared frequencies of each allele.

$$M = \sum_{i=1}^{j} p_i^2$$

For example, let's say we have three allele frequencies, p_1, p_2, and p_3, and want to calculate the overall expected homozygote genotype frequency. First we define the three allele frequencies:

```
> p1 <- 0.2
> p2 <- 0.3
> p3 <- 0.5
```

Then, in order to find the square value of each of these individually, we can use the function `sapply()` to square each one separately. This function is remarkably useful, as you can apply any function you specify to individual elements in a dataset. In this case, we're combining our three p values with `c(...)` and then explicitly stating that we're defining a function (`function(x)`) which is `x^2`.

```
> sapply(c(p1,p2,p3),function(x) x^2)
```

This gives us the value of each p^2 value; however, we want the sum of all those p^2, in which case we just have to wrap this up in a sum function:

```
> sum(sapply(c(p1,p2,p3),function(x) x^2))
```

This gives us an overall homozygote genotype frequency of 38%.

We can then quite easily get an expected heterozygote frequency: since a diploid genotype must either be homozygous or heterozygous, the expected level of heterozygosity is simply one minus homozygosity, or

$$T = 1 - \sum_{i=1}^{j} p_i^2.$$

In our sample above, that means that if our expected level of homozygosity is 0.38, our expected level of heterozygosity is $1 - 0.38$, or 0.62.

Let's read in a real dataset of multiple sampled alleles from Aleppo Pine (*Pinus halepensis*, see Fig. 5.3) in the Eastern Mediterranean, sort through the data, and calculate our expected as well as our observed heterozygote frequencies (adapted from Gershberg et al. 2016). Again, we're assuming the package *popgenr* has already been loaded:

```
> data(genotypes)
```

The data in `genotypes` are all from microsatellites. Microsatellites are segments of DNA characterized by short repeated "blocks" of nucleotide composition (for example, ...[AGT][AGT][AGT][AGT][AGT]...). These types of genetic markers have often been used in research due to the fact that they tend to be highly variable (that is, have high mutation rates).

Let's get a sense of the data with `str()`:

```
> str(genotypes)
'data.frame':    181 obs. of   20 variables:
  $ ID         : Factor w/ 181 levels "1-01","1-02",..:
  $ Pop        : int   1 1 1 1 1 1 1 1 2 2 ...
```

We can see that this data frame has 181 observations (rows) and 20 columns. While eighteen of these columns represent a different locus with an allele designation, where each unique number is a different allele, the first two columns have individual IDs from each sample ($ID) and a population assignment ($Pop). We're going to want to write an iterative code to go through the dataset to make our calculations; to make that easier, let's streamline the data a bit. First, let's make the content of the first column the row names of the data frame, using the function `rownames()`. Row names are a special feature of a dataset, distinct from a regular column, that can be maintained easily while making changes to the rest of the data. Since we're saving column $ID as row names, we can get rid of $ID from the main data frame, and we can also get rid of the $Pop column so that the only columns we have are allele designations:

```
> rownames(genotypes) <- genotypes$ID
> genotypes <- genotypes[,-c(1,2)]
```

The way this dataset is set up, we have two columns for each individual, representing the two copies of one locus in a sampled diploid pine tree. Let's count the total number of loci in the dataset. The `length()` function on a data frame should return only the number of columns. Since each locus is represented by two columns, we can divide that in half to get the total number of loci sampled:

```
> (num.loci <- (length(genotypes))/2)
[1] 9
```

Now we know that we're working with nine different loci. Next we need to figure out how many alleles are actually present at each locus. We will use a `for` loop to perform an allele count `for` each one of our loci. One tricky thing about loops is that as they run they produce variables that by default aren't saved, and in order to capture the output of each iteration you need to have some way in which to save each output into a variable that's "outside" the loop. Let's start by creating a few empty variables that we're going to fill in during our run:

```
> Hom_exp <- NULL
> Het_exp <- NULL
> Hom_obs <- NULL
> Het_obs <- NULL
```

We start our actual loop by specifying that it should last from 1 to the total number of loci (9), and we're going to specify that "n" will be the place holder for each integer in that range

```
> for(n in 1:(num.loci)){
```

This input begins the `for` loop, and now anything we input after the { will be performed `for` all the values in the vector we've specified (from 1 to the total number of loci). Note that nothing we type in after the { will actually work until we eventually close the `for` loop command with a } later in the code. We're going to have to collect each locus as a combination of two columns. To do this, we're first going to collect only half of our range (the odd numbers) into an object "current" so that we can specify a subset that consists of every odd-numbered column plus the one immediately next to it. Remember that the order in the brackets is always row number followed by column number ([row, column]). Leaving row blank but specifying column pulls all the rows of that column, while specifying row and not column pulls all the columns of that row:

```
current <- n*2-1
locus <- c(genotypes[,current], genotypes[,current+1])
alleles <- unique(locus)
```

Often in real multilocus datasets there are situations where there is missing data for certain individuals at certain loci. In this case, missing data is coded as negative one (−1). In this case we don't want to count missing data, so let's remove it from our group of "alleles." We do this by subsetting "alleles" to only those entries which are not −1 using the logical argument not-equal (! =):

```
alleles <- alleles[alleles ! = -1]
```

Now that we have an object containing the alleles at a certain locus, we can start to count how many of each allele there are. To do this, we're actually going to nest another for loop within this loop. We're going to make another variable, p_allele, and we're going to start iterating through the elements in the alleles object we've just made,

```
p_allele <- NULL
for(a in 1:length(alleles)){
```

In this nested loop, we're going to calculate allele frequencies by using an interesting feature of logical operators. When a logical operator returns a FALSE, in R that is considered the equivalent of zero, while when a TRUE is returned it is coded as a one. This means that if you were to sum across a logical operation you would end up with the total number of TRUEs. So we can sum the number of times an element of an object matches (or doesn't match) something in another object and get an effective count of that element in the matched object. Then we can close our nested loop with a }.

```
        p_allele <- c(p_allele,
        sum(alleles[a]==locus) / sum(locus!=-1))
   }
```

At this stage of our loop we're finally at the point where we can calculate our expected homozygous genotype frequency. We do this by using the same `sapply()` function as before, but this time applying it to our newly created "p_allele" object:

```
  Hom_exp <- c(Hom_exp, sum(sapply(p_allele,
        function(x) x^2)))
```

The only thing left to do now is to figure out the observed genotype frequencies for each locus. Let's start by again creating a temporary variable "obs" to keep track of our homozygote counts for each locus. Then we're going to start another nested "for" loop, this time going through all the individuals per column. To do that, we'll specify the range as being from 1 to the number of rows of the dataset (181). We can automatically get the number of rows of any data frame by using the function "nrow."

```
  obs <- 0
  for(i in 1:length(genotypes[,current])){
```

Now we're going to impose conditional statements on our loop. We don't want to estimate homozygosity if there's missing data, so we can use an `if` statement to check every row (in this case "i") in our column ("current") to make sure it doesn't match −1. We're going to immediately follow our first `if` statement which is clearing away the missing data with a nested `if` statement which checks to see if the allele in the first column is the same as the allele in the second column. If that condition is TRUE (that is, homozygote), we finally move on to the command, which in this case is to add 1 to our obs variable:

```
        if(genotypes[i, current]!=-1){
            if(genotypes[i, current]==
                genotypes[i,current+1]){
            obs <- obs+1
            }
        }
    }
```

Once the iteration across the "current" locus is complete, but before we move on to the next one, we want to divide the number of homozygotes at that locus ("obs") by the total number of non-missing genotypes. Just like before, we'll use sum(locus! = -1) to filter out the missing data, but this time we'll divide that value by 2 to represent the number of diploid genotypes or, in other words, individuals:

```
    Hom_obs <- c(Hom_obs, obs/(sum(locus != -1) / 2))
}
```

By inputting that final }, we've now successfully completed our for loop. Let's take a look at the current script in its entirety:

```
for(n in 1:(num.loci)){
    current <- n*2-1
    locus <- c(genotypes[,current],genotypes[,current+1])
    alleles <- unique(locus)
    alleles <- alleles[alleles!=-1]
    p_allele <- NULL
    for(a in 1:length(alleles)){
        p_allele <- c(p_allele,
        sum(alleles[a]==locus)/sum(locus!=-1))
        }
    Hom_exp <- c(Hom_exp, sum(sapply(p_allele,
        function(x) x^2)))
    obs <- 0
    for(i in 1:length(genotypes[,current])){
        if(genotypes[i, current]!=-1){
            if(genotypes[i, current]==
```

```
                    genotypes[i,current+1]){
                    obs <- obs+1
            }
        }
    }
    Hom_obs <- c(Hom_obs,obs/(sum(locus!=-1)/2))
}
```

Now to find the expected and observed heterozygote frequencies we simply subtract our homozygote frequencies from the total sum of our frequencies (1):

```
> Het_exp <- 1 - Hom_exp

> Het_obs <- 1 - Hom_obs
```

Let's plot our observed versus our expected heterozygosity frequencies across these nine loci and see just how well they relate. We'll start by simply using plot of Het_obs and Het_exp, and follow that up with drawing a regression line. We'll use the function lm (linear model) to estimate the linear relationship between the datasets (least squares linear regression), and then we'll wrap that in the function abline, which will draw a straight line on the present plot:

```
> plot(Het_obs, Het_exp)

> abline( lm( Het_exp ~ Het_obs))
```

Looks good, but let's now subset the regression output and print the actual correlation coefficient onto the plot itself. The lm function is quite useful, not just because it can be used to perform linear regressions and ANalysis Of VAriance (ANOVA) calculations, but also because it can be wrapped in the summary function to quickly give us a table of results to manipulate:

```
> reg <- summary(lm(Het_exp ~ Het_obs))
```

```
> print(reg)

> rr <- reg$r.squared

> rrlabel <- paste("r-squared =",round(rr, digits = 3))

> pv <- reg$coefficients[2,4]

> pvlabel <- paste("P-value =",pv)

> text(0.6, 0.2, rrlabel)

> text(0.6, 0.15, pvlabel)
```

Looking at our plot (Fig. 5.4), we should see a pretty good validation that Hardy–Weinberg predictions can be extended to multiple loci and in this case work quite well in predicting a wide range of heterozygosity values.

This process may seem tedious to people that are new to programming. A key part of writing a program is being able to break a task down into

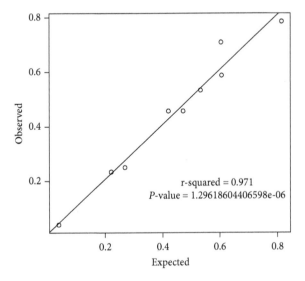

Figure 5.4 Plot of the relationship between observed and expected heterozygote frequencies across nine loci in *Pinus halepensis* trees.

very small individual steps, yet keep organized and understand how these steps fit together in the bigger picture. We tend to intuitively underestimate how many individual steps go into what at first seems like a simple task. However, like any skill this gets easier with practice and the end results are worth it. Keep in mind that you and others can readily reuse this code and *much* larger datasets can be manipulated with ease. Each minute you spend coding is an investment in your future abilities, even if it seems frustrating at the time.

5.3 Blood types and allele frequencies

We've so far mostly discussed allele and genotype frequencies and how we could infer one from the other. But what if you don't know the allele frequencies and only know which phenotypes are present in the population? If you're fortunate enough to know which phenotypes correspond to which genotypes, you can easily estimate the allele frequencies!

Let's consider different blood phenotypes as a simple example. Humans can generally only have one of four major blood types, called *A*, *B*, *AB*, and *O* (let's ignore the + and − rhesus factor and other variants). Each of these corresponds to a certain genotype with alleles *a*, *b*, or *i*: People of blood type *A* can be either *aa* or *ai* genotypes. People with blood type *B* can be either *bb* or *bi* genotypes. Both *A* and *B* are dominant phenotypes to the *O* blood type, and we don't know which ones are homozygotes or heterozygotes. However, a person with blood type *AB* (a codominant phenotype) can only have the *ab* genotype and a person with blood type *O* (a recessive phenotype) can only have the *ii* genotype.

Let's say we're interested in finding out the proportion of *a*, *b*, and *i* alleles. We will use previously determined blood types (phenotypes) of a sample of individuals (Nikolic et al. 2010) and create different objects in R to hold the data:

```
> AB <- 5
> A <- 30
```

```
> B <- 7
> O <- 36
```

Let's save the total number of individuals sampled:

```
> (N <- AB + A + B + O)
[1] 78
```

The phenotype proportions in our sample can then be found by dividing the number of each blood type by the total number of individuals (N):

```
> A/N
[1] 0.3846154
> B/N
[1] 0.08974359
> AB/N
[1] 0.06410256
> O/N
[1] 0.4615385
```

So about 38% of the sample had the *A* blood type phenotype, about 9% were blood type *B*, only about 6% had the *AB* blood type, and approximately 46% were blood type *O*. This doesn't seem to tell us much about the total frequencies of the *a*, *b*, and *i* alleles by themselves, but finding the phenotype proportions is a good first step. Remember the expected genotype calculation based on the Hardy–Weinberg proportions? We already know that *O* blood types can only have the *ii* genotypes, and based on the Hardy–Weinberg predictions we expect that the number of *ii* genotypes should be the squared value of the underlying *i* allele frequency (p_i^2). So then the assumed *i* allele frequency (p_i) is simply the square root of the total proportion of the *ii* genotypes:

```
> (Pi <- sqrt(O/N))
[1] 0.6793662
```

Note that we're just starting by focusing on the *O* phenotype, and that while the *A* and *B* phenotypes also contain some proportion of the *i* alleles as *ai* and *bi* heterozygotes, our theoretically expected number of *ii* homozygotes is not going to be affected by the fact that there are two more alleles "hiding" *i* alleles as heterozygotes. Remember that we're assuming that all the conditions of the Hardy–Weinberg assumption are at play (for example, fully random association of alleles), so the theoretical proportions still hold true. So now we at least know that the expected allele frequency of the *i* allele in our sample is about 68%. This gives us a starting point to begin figuring out the *a* and *b* allele frequencies. We can set up the same equation here to see how we can get the frequency of all the individuals of genotypes *aa*, *ai* (phenotype A), and *ii* (phenotype O).

So if we want to solve the equation for our blood type allele frequencies, which once again we're assuming is properly represented by the Hardy–Weinberg proportions, we're going to need p_a as well as p_i. Working backwards, our equation

$$p_a^2 + 2 * (p_a * p_i) + p_i^2$$

becomes

$$(p_a + p_i)^2.$$

And because we know that this value is just the total proportion of *A* and *O* blood types in the sample, we can use the phenotype values we've gathered to find it:

$$(p_a + p_i)^2 = \frac{A + O}{N}.$$

We can rearrange this to

$$p_a + p_i = \sqrt{\frac{A + O}{N}},$$

and from here it's easy to get p_a:

$$p_a = \sqrt{\frac{A + O}{N}} - p_i.$$

```
> (Pa <- sqrt((A+O)/N)-Pi)
[1]  0.2405
```

Now we can do just the same but with p_b:

```
> (Pb <- sqrt((B+O)/N)-Pi)
[1]  0.06311748
```

What do these proportions add up to? Let's see.

```
> Pa + Pb + Pi
[1]  0.9829837
```

This should give you a value quite close to one, but not exactly. Let's change the accuracy:

```
> signif(Pa + Pb + Pi, 1)
[1]  1
```

The `signif()` function here only displays the answer to the significant figures specified after the comma.

This should be unsatisfying; we don't want to try to resort to a trick to force the sum to come out to one, which is what we know it should be. The problem is that the phenotype frequencies are deviating slightly from what they would be under true Hardy–Weinberg predictions, and we are not taking this "tension" fully into account when we solve for the allele frequencies bit by bit, independently of the whole. To help illustrate, here is the predicted number of *AB* heterozygotes based on our allele frequency estimates.

```
> N*2*Pa*Pb
[1]  2.368042
```

Yet the observed number was more than twice this value. We can do better and write an algorithm to modify these estimates to a maximum-likelihood solution based on the entire observed dataset simultaneously.

5.4 Expectation Maximization algorithm

Algorithm is a term most people are familiar with, but struggle to readily define. The word actually comes from the name of the ninth-century mathematician Muḥammad ibn Mūsā al-Khwārizmī (al-Khwārizmī was latinized as *Algorismus*), who also gave us the word "algebra" (the Arabic *al-jabr* means to "rejoin" or "complete"). A very simple definition is that an algorithm is just a series of operations executed in a specific order.

Algorithms are pretty standard in most quantitative disciplines, and recently types of algorithms termed "machine learning" have been applied to population genetics inferences. Machine learning has recently become a hot topic in many data analysis circles and is often treated as a brand new approach. However, many classically employed methods focus on precisely the same concept as machine learning; that is, the continual updating of information to reach more accurate conclusions. One approach that does this is called the Expectation Maximization (EM) algorithm.

Earlier, in our blood type example, we were able to calculate what genotypes we'd expect to see, given the size of our samples and assuming that we are in Hardy–Weinberg equilibrium. In the following calculations, there will be a fair number of parentheses showing up. Make sure that there are as many open parentheses, "(," as there are closed parentheses, ")," in every input. Missing one of these can be the bane of programmers' existence, as everything you've input can stop dead in its tracks for no obvious reason until every orphaned parenthesis is resolved.

```
> (Paa <- A*(Pa^2/((Pa^2)+2*(Pa*Pi))))
 [1] 4.511539
> (Pai <- A*(2*(Pa*Pi))/((Pa^2)+(2*(Pa*Pi))))
 [1] 25.48846
> (Pbb <- B*(Pb^2/((Pb^2)+(2*(Pb*Pi)))))
 [1] 0.3107377
> (Pbi <- B*(2*(Pb*Pi))/((Pb^2)+(2*(Pb*Pi))))
 [1] 6.689262
```

```
> (Pii <- O)
 [1]  36
> (Pab <- AB)
 [1]  5
```

Now we re-estimate the allele frequencies from these Hardy–Weinberg proportions.

```
> (Pa <-  ((2*Paa)+Pai+Pab)/(2*N))
 [1]  0.2532791
> (Pb <-  ((2*Pbb)+Pbi+Pab)/(2*N))
 [1]  0.07891499
> (Pi <-  ((2*Pii)+Pai+Pbi)/(2*N))
 [1]  0.6678059
```

Then we can feed these frequencies back into our genotype estimations:

```
> (Paa <- A*(Pa^2/((Pa^2)+(2*(Pa*Pi)))))
 [1]  4.782187
> (Pai <- A*(2*(Pa*Pi))/((Pa^2)+(2*(Pa*Pi))))
 [1]  25.21781
> (Pbb <- B*(Pb^2/((Pb^2)+(2*(Pb*Pi)))))
 [1]  0.3905227
> (Pbi <- B*(2*(Pb*Pi))/((Pb^2)+(2*(Pb*Pi))))
 [1]  6.609477
```

We can then re-estimate the allele frequencies again and again until we converge on the maximum-likelihood values of the allele frequencies. This would all be a lot simpler if we could write a function which kept running this feedback until the values were similar enough to the previous estimate to be considered effectively unchanged. Let's start from the beginning and make all this into one function. Just to be safe, let's clear all our saved variables.

```
> rm(list = ls())
```

The function `rm()` removes whatever objects you give it, and `ls()` lists all the objects saved in your R session environment. Now, with a fresh slate, enter in the observed data again.

```
> AB <- 5
> A <- 30
> B <- 7
> O <- 36
> N <- AB + A + B + O
```

We estimate the allele frequencies just as before:

```
> Pi <- sqrt(O/N)
> Pa <- sqrt((A + O)/N) - Pi
> Pb <- sqrt((B + O)/N) - Pi
```

Now we can start putting together the actual function to help us with our maximum-likelihood estimation.

As an example, a very simple function can be defined and called like so:

```
> SQUARE <- function(q) q^2
> SQUARE(5)
[1] 25
```

We defined a function named SQUARE to take in a value (q) and square it. When we called SQUARE() with 5 it returned 25, which is probably correct, so congratulations! You've written an R function!

Let's open up a new R script and begin typing out our expected allele frequency function. We'll start by making some place-holder variables for our updated allele frequencies. (Note that the "0"s below are zeros and not the letter O.)

```
> Pi0 <- 0
> Pa0 <- 0
> Pb0 <- 0
> counter <- 0
```

We'll want to name our function something informative, so let's call our function EM, for Expectation Maximization:

```
> EM <- function(Pi, Pa, Pb){
```

We have to specify how many variables can be read by our function. In this case we state that three variables (initial values of `Pi`, `Pa`, and `Pb`) will be expected when our function is called. Notice the open brace "{" at the end of the function declaration. Braces delimit all the commands that will go into the function. Our function is going to keep iterating for as long as it takes for us to converge on a value. To do this, we'll use a `while` loop. This type of loop is very similar to the `for` loop we've been using, but instead of specifying a vector for the loop to go through we'll give it a specific "exit" condition that will mark the end of the loop. In fact, by using the logical operator "&&" we can string together any number of conditions that will keep the iterations coming until all our conditions are met. In this case, we'll set our exit condition to be the convergence of each of our previous values with our updated estimates, with convergence defined as the point when our new estimates (`Pi`, `Pa`, `Pb`) are identical to the last estimates in the iteration (`Pi0`, `Pa0`, `Pb0`):

```
while((round(Pi0,12)  == round(Pi,12))==FALSE &&
      (round(Pa0,12)  == round(Pa,12))==FALSE &&
      (round(Pb0,12)  == round(Pb,12))==FALSE) {
```

So as soon as all three of those conditions return a `TRUE`, our loop will end. Next in the function we save the new iterations as our next batch of old iterations:

```
Pi0 <- Pi
Pa0 <- Pa
Pb0 <- Pb
```

Now we calculate our expected genotype frequencies from the allele frequencies:

```
Paa <- A*(Pa0^2/((Pa0^2)+(2*(Pa0*Pi0)))))
Pai <- A*(2*(Pa0*Pi0))/((Pa0^2)+(2*(Pa0*Pi0)))
Pbb <- B*(Pb0^2/((Pb0^2)+(2*(Pb0*Pi0)))))
Pbi <- B*(2*(Pb0*Pi0))/((Pb0^2)+(2*(Pb0*Pi0)))
Pii <- O
Pab <- AB
```

Finally, we calculate our new estimates of our allele frequencies:

```
(Pa <- ((2*Paa)+Pai+Pab)/(2*N))
(Pb <- ((2*Pbb)+Pbi+Pab)/(2*N))
(Pi <- ((2*Pii)+Pai+Pbi)/(2*N))
```

Since the parentheses around each calculation specify that the results are to be printed as they finish, we can use these as a good visual cue to make sure our function is actually running. It would be interesting to keep track of just how many loops our iteration goes through before our conditions are met. Before we close our `while` loop with a closed brace, we'll add one to our counter variable (which started at zero) so that by the end of all our iterations we'll have the total number of loops saved as a variable:

```
    counter <- counter+1
}
```

Now the `while` loop will keep running within the confines of the braces until all the conditions are met, at which point R will be able to read past those confines and look for the next closed brace to mark the end of the function. Before we conclude our function, though, we'll want to report what we actually found from all those iterations. To do that, we'll specify what should be our end product by using the `return()` function:

```
    return(c(paste("Pi =",Pi, ", Pa =", Pa, ",
    Pb=", Pb, ", Number of loops =", counter)))
}
```

We've now specified that after the loop our function should return a pasted-together text specifying our maximum-likelihood estimation, as well as the number of loops we went through to converge on our answer. Our final closed brace marks the end of the function. Now let's run our function and compare the EM output with our original estimates of the allele frequencies:

```
> c(Pi, Pa, Pb) # Our initial estimates
[1] 0.67936622 0.24049999 0.06311748
> EM(Pi,Pa,Pb)
[1] "Pi = 0.66522628... , Pa = 0.25532200... ,
    Pb = 0.07945172... , Number of loops = 12"
```

So after twelve iterations we've converged on allele frequency values that, unlike our initial estimates, actually sum to one.

```
> 0.66522628 + 0.25532200 + 0.07945172
[1] 1
```

Even if we have arbitrary starting allele frequencies, such as $p_i = p_a = p_b = 1/3$, the algorithm should still quickly converge to these same values.

Until now we've mostly focused on datasets from fixed time points and have primarily been comparing samples of allele frequencies to predictions based on an infinitely large theoretical population. In the next chapter we'll start looking at finite populations and changes in allele frequencies over time.

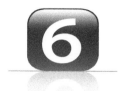

Genetic Variation

⊣ Term Definitions ⊢

Continuous time: Time that flows continuously without occurring in units.

Diffusion: A passive net movement of particles from a region of high concentration to (a) region(s) of lower concentration.

Discrete time: Time that is broken into units, such as generations.

Genetic drift: Change in allele frequency by evolutionary sampling error.

Factorial: The product of all positive integers less than or equal to a starting positive interger and represented by an ! (for example, $4! = 4 \times 3 \times 2 \times 1 = 24$).

Transition probability: A probability of changing from one state to another (or remaining in the same state). These are usually organized into a matrix of all possible states.

6.1 Genetic drift and evolutionary sampling

A key idea upon which much of computational population genetics rests is that the vast majority of expected genetic variation observed in populations will be due to seemingly random changes and not because of direct evolutionary selection. The basic idea is simple enough: Organisms sometimes die or don't reproduce by random chance, while other organisms may produce more offspring than average by chance, and that affects what

Population Genetics with R: An Introduction for Life Scientists. Áki J. Láruson and Floyd A. Reed, Oxford University Press (2021). © Áki J. Láruson & Floyd A. Reed.
DOI: 10.1093/oso/9780198829539.003.0006

genetic variants pass down through generations. One of the founders of the Population Genetics discipline, Sewall Wright, referred to this back in 1929 as allele frequencies appearing to "drift" from one frequency to another over the generations, without a steady direction toward becoming fixed or extinct in the population. The term "genetic drift" has stuck. The idea that neutral variants, and not variants explicitly driven by natural selection, made up the majority of the genetic variation observed was first formalized by Motoo Kimura in the sixties and remains a key consideration for statistical analyses of observed genetic variation in populations. The significance of the theory of neutral variation is that it provides a succinct expectation for observed genetic variation, and therefore provides a concise null hypothesis against which to test alternative hypotheses. Much like in Chapter 4, when we made a series of assumptions to predict the interactions between allele and genotype frequencies, in order to quantitatively approach the random changes in allele frequencies over time there are generally a lot of assumptions that have to be made regarding several factors at play. For example, how exactly do variants get passed down through the generations? What about the occurrence of new mutations and migration bringing in new variants? There are just about an infinite amount of considerations that could be made, but in order to make this manageable we're going to assume just a few simple facts:

1. Generations of organisms do not overlap (one generation dies as the next emerges).
2. Organisms are diploid (each individual has two copies of their genome).
3. There's a fixed population size, (N), which does not change across generations.
4. Each allele is "drawn" at random, independent of all other alleles, from the previous generation to pass on to the next.

These assumptions are what make up the Wright–Fisher model of genetic drift. Using the assumptions inherent to this model, we can attempt to predict patterns we might observe of neutrally changing variants being inherited across multiple generations. The last stipulation of the Wright–Fisher model above is that any one allele is not more likely to be drawn than any other allele. This is what defines neutrality—there is no positive or negative selection occurring. This may seem overly constrained, as we know fitness differences exist in some cases, but keep in mind that drift *always* exists and affects alleles under selection as well as neutral variants, so drift is critically important to understand. One direct computational way to approach the expected change in allele composition occurring every generation is to think of inheritance primarily in terms of probabilities.

It's generally assumed when discussing probabilities that there is an underlying distribution for how probable or improbable some event is. Using the right distribution of probabilities across different observations (quantiles) is critical. In the previous chapter we were working with the χ^2 distribution to compare observations across specific categories. Here we are going to use a binomial distribution to work with collections of binary outcomes. A binary event is an event that either occurred or didn't occur—like when flipping a coin, it's either heads or tails—and it can be quite useful to think of alleles in this manner.

Let's say we have a very small population of five diploid individuals made up of two alleles—one allele is present as three copies (black circles) and the other is present as seven copies (white circles). If we randomly draw circles to make up the next generation, the chance of drawing a black allele is 3/10 and the chance of a white allele is 7/10.

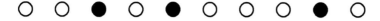

Assuming all copies have an equal chance of reproducing, what is the chance that the next generation, kept at the same size of ten, will be exactly the same as before, with just three copies of the black allele and seven copies of the white allele? This result depends on the black allele being sampled three times and the white allele being sampled seven times.

```
> 0.3^3 * 0.7^7
[1] 0.002223566
```

That's a pretty small chance: about 0.2%. However, this equation is incomplete because there are actually a lot of different ways to end up with a pattern of three black and seven white alleles. The first three could be black and the last seven white, or the first, third, and fifth black and the rest white, etc. The total number of combinations can be calculated using factorials:

$$\binom{n = 10}{k = 3} = \frac{n!}{k!(n-k)!} = \frac{10!}{3!7!} = 120.$$

So there are a total of 120 ways that we could possibly get three black and seven white alleles from sampling the original population. This operation can be referred to as "ten choose three," because we've calculated all the ways to choose three "successes" out of ten "attempts." We can calculate this in R using the choose function:

```
> choose(10, 3)
[1] 120
```

So now our full equation for the probability of exactly three black and seven white alleles showing up in the next generation becomes

$$P(3 \text{ and } 7) = 120 \times 0.3^3 \times 0.7^7 \approx 0.267$$

```
> 120 * 0.3^3 * 0.7^7
[1] 0.2668279
```

That suggests there's a much higher chance than we originally calculated (from 0.02% to over 26%) of keeping the same proportions from one generation to the next. What we are really talking about here is the binomial probability

$$P(k \text{ out of } n) = \binom{n}{k} p^k (1-p)^{(n-k)},$$

where n is the total sample size (10 in our example), k is the number of observed variants we're interested in (3), and p is the frequency of that type (0.3).

So in this small population there is about a one-in-four chance that the allele frequency stays the same in the next generation. Turning this around, there is about a three-in-four chance that it *will* change in the next generation. In statistics we expect that when we take a sample, the frequency in the sample is often not exactly the same as in the original population we are drawing from. However, the larger the sample, the smaller we expect the deviation to be by chance. Genetic drift is essentially evolutionary sampling error, and the deviations between generations are greater in smaller populations (that is, smaller samples).

We can also readily calculate the extreme cases: that the next generation will be made up of all black or all white alleles. Intuitively we can predict that the probability of sampling all white alleles is larger than all black, because of the frequency difference. The probability of getting all white alleles in the next generation is $0.7^{10} \approx 0.028$. Note that there is only one way to get this result: all copies have to be white, so we don't have to worry about the n choose k binomial coefficient. The probability of all black alleles by random chance is $0.3^{10} \approx 5.9 \times 10^{-6}$. So from our example starting point we don't expect complete fixation or loss of one allele or the other in a single generation, but more likely than not it will change in frequency due to no forces other than random sampling.

Let's consider a single locus in a diploid organism where a mutation has occurred, giving us the possibility of two alleles existing there: A and a. We can compose a matrix containing all the possible genotypes that are possible with just two alleles. Remember that we are assuming this organism is diploid (again this is an often-used assumption, but there are plenty of exceptions), so we then expect there to be a grand total of three distinct genotypes possible: AA, Aa, and aa.

The first thing we're going to do is save the number of individuals we're dealing with as an object (N), and then we'll figure out how many copies of the allele A are possible, given our number of individuals. The number of possible copies should just be a vector ranging from zero (the allele is extinct) to two times (remember, diploid) the number of individuals (2*N), at which point the allele is fixed in the population:

```
> N <- 1 #One diploid individual
> possible <- 0:(2*N) #Number of possible copies of an allele
```

We can now draw the binomial probability (P) of having a particular copy number (k), given a certain allele frequency (p) and the total copy numbers possible (n):

$$P(k|p, n) = \binom{n}{k}p^k(1 - p)^{n-k}.$$

So if we start with one copy of A we have the following transition probabilities in the next generation:

Copies Next Generation	0	1	2
Binomial Probability	1/4	1/2	1/4

So the most likely outcome (50%) is that we'll stay at one copy of A, but we have a 25% chance of either losing or gaining a copy of A in the next generation.

We're setting up our framework here looking at a small test case (one autogamic individual!) so that we can easily expand our code later to handle the rapidly increasing complexity that comes with adding more individuals. Let's use the R function dbinom to get our binomial probabilities for each of our possible allele counts, given all possible starting frequencies. We'll save these binomial probabilities as object P and then create a matrix containing these values that we'll call Q:

```
> P <- NULL #Vector to hold our probabilities
> for(i in possible){
    P <- c(P,dbinom(possible, size=2*N, prob=i/(2*N)))
}
> (Q <- matrix(P, ncol=2*N+1, byrow=T)) #Arrange into matrix
        [,1] [,2] [,3]
```

```
[1,] 1.00   0.0 0.00
[2,] 0.25   0.5 0.25
[3,] 0.00   0.0 1.00
```

We now have a transition probability matrix that describes what to expect, given all possible starting states. Each row shows us the probability of transitioning from zero, one, or two copies of *A* (going down the matrix), to zero, one, or two copies, respectively across the columns, in a subsequent generation. Notice that in the top row, where we're assuming that we have zero copies of *A*, we're seeing a 100% probability of staying at zero copies. And similarly, in the bottom row, we see a 100% chance of staying at two copies of *A* in the next generation. These should make sense, thinking about extinction and fixation within the confines of our model. We're assuming that no new mutations are arising that disrupt our fixed state, so once the *A* allele has saturated the population it'll never be anything but fixed. Similarly, if the *A* goes extinct it can never again arise, and will stay at zero forever. This is not very realistic, since we know that new mutations arise and even lost mutations can potentially re-emerge, but once again we're sacrificing immobilizing realism for functional reductionism.

If we assume that every generation these transition probabilities hold, then the only thing changing generation to generation is the starting frequency. So across the generations the probability of our allele *A* ending at a certain copy number is the composite probability of the transition seen in each previous generation. The probability of *A* being lost in three generations could be visualized like so:

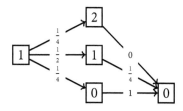

Because we assume that what happens in each generation is independent of what happens in any other generation, we can multiply the probabilities along any one path to get the cumulative probability of the allele following that particular path (probability multiplication rule). So the probability that the A allele stayed as one copy and then went extinct is just

$$\frac{1}{2} * \frac{1}{4} = \frac{1}{8} = 12.5\%.$$

But what if we want the total probability of A going extinct in three generations, regardless of what path it went through? Because each hypothetical path is mutually exclusive of all other paths (that is, there's no way for an allele to simultaneously experience more than one path in a single generation), we can add up all the cumulative probabilities of each path (the probability addition rule):

$$\left(\frac{1}{4} * 0\right) + \left(\frac{1}{2} * \frac{1}{4}\right) + \left(\frac{1}{4} * 1\right) = \frac{3}{8} = 37.5\%.$$

Next let's create a matrix object that gives us a starting state. In order to set it up like our transition matrix, we're going to have each column represent one of our three possible transition states (zero, one, and two copies), but we're only going to need one row in this matrix. Let's first generate the matrix object x with all probabilities set to zero, which we can easily update later:

```
> (x <- matrix(c(rep(0,2*N+1)), ncol=2*N+1, byrow=T))
      [,1] [,2] [,3]
[1,]   0    0    0
```

Now let's assume we're starting with a single copy of A, which means we'll set the probability in the "one copy" column (the second column) to 100%:

```
> x[,2] <- 1
> x
      [,1] [,2] [,3]
[1,]   0    1    0
```

We can now use matrix multiplication to get all our transition probabilities, given our starting state. This should give us the exact same probabilities we worked out earlier for a single generation transition. Refer back to Chapter 3 if you need a refresher on matrix multiplication in R.

```
> (R <- x%*%Q)
      [,1] [,2] [,3]
[1,] 0.25  0.5 0.25
```

Now let's visualize our transition probabilities over multiple generations. Let's start with assigning some color and shape variables that we'll be using consistently, set our generation variable g to start at one for each of our transition states, and then plot our first-generation transition probabilities with an accompanying legend. We're going to use a couple of neat features of the legend function by specifying our placement with "bottom-left." This would normally plop our legend down in the expected bottom left-hand corner of our plot, but we're going to set xpd to TRUE and specify an inset command, which should place our legend on the *top* left side of our plot. Effectively what we're doing is allowing the legend to have its own location parameters outside of the plot provided (xpd = TRUE), and saying that we want to move it up the y-axis by the full length of our figure margin (inset=c(0,1)). Finally, we'll specify that we don't want a box around our legend by specifying bty="n."

```
> color <- c("brown","blue","grey")

> shape <- c(15,19,17)

> #Start with generation 1 for all states
> g <- rep(1,ncol(R))

> plot(points(x=NULL, xlim=c(1,10), ylim=c(0,1),
    ylab="Probability",
    xlab="Generations")
```

```
> legend("bottomleft",
    legend=c("Extinct","One copy","Fixed"),
    col=color, pch=shape,
    xpd=TRUE, inset=c(0,1), bty="n")
```

Now that we've set up our canvas, let's fill in our transition probabilities by creating a short `while` loop, where each loop updates the probabilities and adds one to our generation time. Let's also set our exit condition to be when g reaches ten generations. Note that since we can't set a condition based on multiple elements in a vector, we can set the condition explicitly so that as long as the first element of g is less than 10 (g[1] < 10) our loop will continue to run:

```
> while(g[1]<=10){
    (R <- R%*%Q)
    g <- g+1
    points(g, R, col=color, pch=shape)
}
```

Taking a look at our output from the above code, it should look similar to Fig. 6.1. We can see that the probability of A staying as a single copy drops pretty quickly from 0.5 to practically zero within just a handful of generations. Notice that the "Fixed" and "Extinct" conditions (which perfectly overlap) pretty quickly rise to the same probability as the starting frequency of the allele. Remember that little detail; we'll revisit that a bit later.

Try changing the starting condition by manipulating x so that we start off with A being fixed in the population,

$$x = \begin{pmatrix} 0 & 0 & 1 \end{pmatrix},$$

or with A being extinct:

$$x = \begin{pmatrix} 1 & 0 & 0 \end{pmatrix}.$$

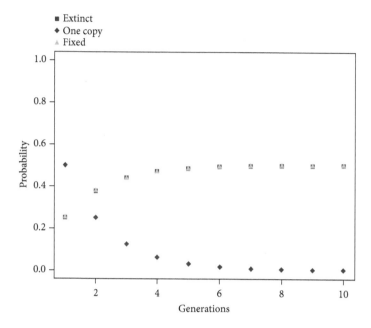

Figure 6.1 Probability of an allele existing at a certain copy number over generational time. Assumes binomial probability of a change in state, representing random fluctuation, and that the allele started as a single copy in a population of one diploid individual.

What do you see when you plot the results of these starting conditions? What you should be seeing is that if you start an allele off being fixed or extinct, it's going to stay in that condition, no matter how long you run your loop. Hence fixation and extinction are *absorbing boundaries* in this model: once you become fixed or go extinct there's no coming back.

A quick word of warning regarding while loops: it can be quite easy to mess up an exit condition for a while loop so that you never actually meet your condition. This will result in your code running indefinitely and is generally not a good use of anyone's time. If you ever find yourself in a loop limbo, you can either press the red "stop sign" that shows up in the upper right-hand corner of your terminal screen if you're using RStudio, or you can press CTRL and C on your keyboard if you're running R directly on the command line.

Now let's expand our code to something a little more interesting. Let's consider a small population of ten diploid individuals (so a total of twenty loci in the population) that again will start with a single *A* allele cropping up in one individual. We should have twenty-one possible states, since we're always including "zero copies" as our first state. Let's alter our code slightly to account for the multiple intermediate frequencies that can now be possible between the "Fixed" and "Extinct" states:

```
> N <- 10 #Ten diploid individual
> possible <- 0:(2*N) #Number of possible copies of an allele

> P <- NULL #Vector to hold our probabilities
> for(i in possible){
    P <- c(P,dbinom(possible, size=2*N, prob=i/(2*N)))
}

> #Our transition matrix should be 21 rows by 21 columns
> Q <- matrix(P, ncol=2*N+1, byrow=T)

> #Create our starting state matrix
> x <- matrix(c(rep(0,2*N+1)), ncol=2*N+1, byrow=T)

> x[2] <- 1 #Set the prob. of starting with one copy to 100%

> R <- x%*%Q #Get our first gen. transition probabilities

> #Change our color and shape parameters to include
    all the entries between our first "Extinct" state,
    and our final "Fixed" state
> color <- c("brown", rep("blue",ncol(R)-2),"grey")
> shape <- c(15, rep(19,ncol(R)-2), 17)

> #Start with generation 1 for all states
> g <- rep(1,ncol(R))

> #Let's increase our x-axis range to 100
> plot(points(x=NULL, xlim=c(1,100), ylim=c(0,1),
    ylab="Probability",
```

```
     xlab="Generations")

> #The unique() function avoids replicates for color & shape
> legend("bottomleft",
     legend=c("Extinct","Intermediate","Fixed"),
     col=unique(color), pch=unique(shape),
     inset=c(0,1), xpd=TRUE, bty="n")

> while(g[1]<100){
     R <- R%*%Q
     g <- g+1
     points(g, R, col=color, pch=shape)
}

> #Finally let's add two horizontal lines to our plot:
> #The starting allele frequency of A
> abline(h=1/(2*N), lwd=2)
> #And the starting allele frequency of a
> abline(h=1-(1/(2*N)), lwd=2, col="orange", lty=2)
```

From this you should hopefully be seeing something like Fig. 6.2. Notice that the probability of fixation (gray triangles) seems to be reaching an asymptote located at the starting allele frequency of A. The fixation probability appears to increase quite slowly and levels off at a probability of 5%. On the other hand, the probability of going extinct (red squares) seems to increase quite quickly and levels off at 95%! This makes some sense: we're saying that there's a random chance of increasing or decreasing in frequency every generation, and if we start with only one copy of an allele, the probability of that one allele still just drifting around the population in 100 generations is going to be pretty slim. Actually, there is an important point here hiding in plain sight. The rarer allele started off at a frequency of 1/20 and after several generations arrived at a probability of fixation of $0.05 = 1/20$. Let's see what happens when we start changing our starting allele frequency. Re-run the code where we set our initial copy number, and this time let's say that half of all our individuals have the A allele (an A allele frequency of 50%):

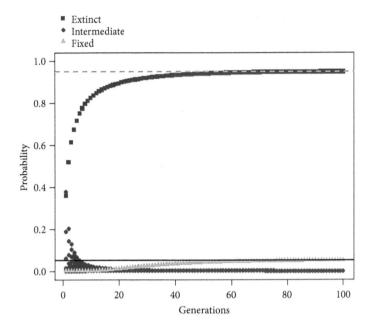

Figure 6.2 Probability of an allele state over generational time in a twenty-locus model. Starting allele frequency ($p = 5\%$) is shown with a solid black line, $1-p$ is shown with a dashed orange line.

```
> x <- matrix(c(rep(0,2*N+1)), ncol=2*N+1, byrow=T)

> x[11] <- 1 #Set the prob. of starting at ten copies to 100%
```

Now re-run the rest of the code to see our transition probabilities when half of all our loci have the *A* allele. You should be seeing something similar to Fig. 6.3. There appears to be a much more gradual increase in the probability of going extinct, as well as in the probability of becoming fixed. Once again, notice that the fixation probability levels off exactly at our starting allele frequency of 50%, and so too does our extinction probability. Under neutral genetic drift, the probability of ultimate fixation of an allele is equal to its starting frequency in the population. For brand new mutations this probability is $1/(2N)$.

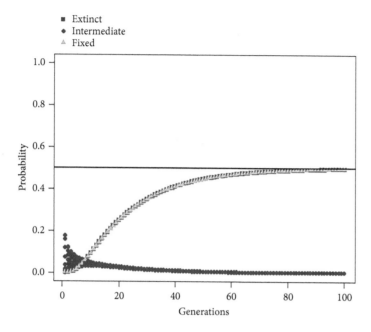

Figure 6.3 Probability of an allele state across generations when starting allele frequency is equal to 50%.

In fact, notice that this plot looks a bit similar to our first probability plot where we only had a single individual. Let's take a look at those side by side (Fig. 6.4). Both of these have the same starting allele frequency of 50%, but the difference is the total number of loci (individuals) in our model. In our first case of the single individual, our probabilities of fixing or going extinct reach their peak frequencies within the first ten generations, while in the larger population it takes almost 100 generations for those probabilities to fully flatten.

This suggests something about the effect of population size on maintenance of alleles that are subject to genetic drift. We're thinking about alleles as being sampled from one generation to make up the next. Genetic drift is the observation of small changes in the proportion of alleles that result from sampling error. Just like with statistical sampling error, large samples (large populations) have smaller sampling errors; that is, smaller

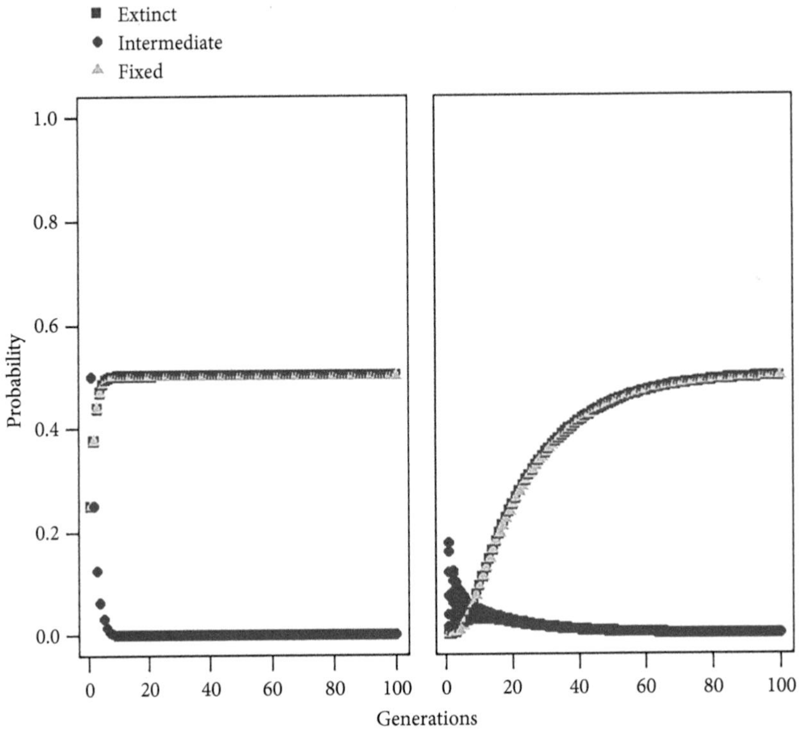

Figure 6.4 Probability of an allele state across generations when starting allele frequency is equal to 50%. Comparing single-diploid individual (left) with ten-diploid individuals (right).

overall changes in allele frequency in each generation. What makes these changes "neutral" is that the observed change is apparently random and without direction. Once again, we have to reiterate that this is a comparatively simplistic model of genetic change over time which makes a lot of simplifying assumptions about the real interplay between selection on individual genetic elements and the stochastic nature of demography across generations.

Despite this inherent randomness, theory allows us to come up with some general rules of thumb (we'll touch on the methods behind these rules in later chapters). For example, it takes about $4 \times N$ generations for a new mutation to reach fixation if we take it as a given that it will eventually fix. Also, after about N generations, we can assume that an allele has undergone so much drift that it can essentially be at any frequency (it has "forgotten" its starting point). Finally, we assume that neutral variation will not tend to hang around for long. An allele usually reaches loss or fixation in less than $3N$ generations even when starting from an intermediate frequency (much less if close to a frequency of zero or one). While studies that quantify variation over many generations in a controlled setting are difficult, expensive, and therefore exceedingly rare, let's take a look at at least one real dataset of allele frequency changes over multiple generations.

6.2 Variation over time

One of the benchmark empirical studies of the phenomenon of genetic drift was provided by the hero of early genetics: the vinegar fly *Drosophila melanogaster* (they are most often called "fruit flies," but very pedantic entomologists will say that name should belong to the family Tephritidae).

In the fifties, Peter Buri conducted the amazingly laborious experiment of independently evolving over 100 small groups of *D. melanogaster* flies with mutant eye-color phenotypes for twenty generations. He started each group of sixteen flies at a 50% frequency for two *bw* ("brown") alleles, which gave homozygous (bw^{75}/bw^{75}, using his original notation) individuals bright red-orange eyes, while heterozygous (bw^{75}/bw) individuals were distinguishable by noticeably lighter orange eyes. Flies that were not carrying the bw^{75} allele (*bw/bw* homozygotes) would show up with white eyes. To keep the population size constant, in each generation a new group of sixteen flies was drawn randomly from the offspring of the previous generation to serve as the next group of parents. By looking at eye color, Buri counted the shifts in copy numbers of bw^{75} over time across over 100 replicates, and this whole thing was done twice!

Before we take a look at Buri's data, let's first visualize our earlier simulations in a new way so we can more easily compare it. Let's simulate a scenario that follows Buri's experiment by setting our population size to sixteen individuals. Then let's modify our `while` loop slightly so that we're no longer plotting points on a graph, but instead saving the transition probabilities for each new generation in a matrix called `Prob`. We'll do this by using the function `rbind` to bind together each new output as a new row in our matrix:

```
> N <- 16 #Our 16 diploid individuals
> possible <- 0:(2*N) #32 possible sites in the population

> #Create our starting state matrix
> x <- matrix(c(rep(0,2*N+1)), ncol=2*N+1, byrow=T)

> x[N+1] <- 1 #Give half our individuals the eye color allele

> P <- NULL #Vector to hold our probabilities
> for(i in possible){
     P <- c(P,dbinom(possible, size=2*N, prob=i/(2*N)))
}

> #This time our transition matrix is 33 rows by 33 columns
> Q <- matrix(P, ncol=2*N+1, byrow=T)

> R <- x%*%Q #Get our first gen. transition probabilities

>#Start our new matrix with our first generation output
> Prob <- R

> #Start with generation 1 for all states
> g <- rep(1,ncol(R))

> #In the loop below, you can simply comment out the
     points function by putting a # in front of it
> while(g[1]<19){ #Change our generation run to 19
     R <- R%*%Q
     Prob <- rbind(Prob,R) #Update our matrix
     g <- g+1
     #points(g, R, col=color, pch=shape)
}
```

Now we have a filled in matrix, `Prob`, that has our transition probabilities across generations. Let's compare these probabilities with the actual observed counts of allele bw^{75}. Instead of visualizing our output like before, let's visualize our output in three dimensions so that our extinct and fixed states don't overlap on our plot. To do this, we'll use the persp function to plot not just our generations and transition probabilities, but our number of alleles as well. In the code below we'll create a 3D plot from simulation data, then read in the observation values from Buri's 1956 paper describing the experiment and plot those data in the same way.

```
> persp(x = 1:g[1], #The range of generations
        y = possible, #Number of alleles possible in the model
        z = Prob, #Matrix of probabilities
        theta = 60, phi = 20, #Adjust to rotate the view
        xlab = "Generations", ylab = "Number of alleles",
        zlab = "Probability",
        shade = 0.3 #Adjust shading of surface
)

#Read in the data from Buri 1956
> data(fly)

> persp(x = 1:g[1],
        y = possible,
        z = fly[-1,], #Matrix of observations,
        omitting first row starting state
        theta = 60, phi = 20,
        xlab = "Generations", ylab = "Number of alleles",
        zlab = "Observations",
        shade = 0.3
)
```

If you want these two plots to be on the same figure, you can actually specify that you want R to arrange a certain number of plots either beside each other, above each other, or arranged in a multiple plot array. To do this, you can use our old friend the par function. *Before* running your plot generating code, you can specify how many columns and rows you want to arrange your plots into by specifying those in the argument mfrow. For example, if you want to plot our two earlier figures side by side, you can specify that you want upcoming plots to be arranged into a single row with two columns by running the following code before everything else:

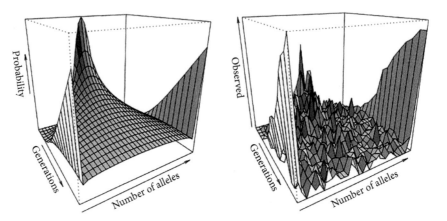

Figure 6.5 Comparison of binomial transition probabilities in a model of sixteen diploid individuals over twenty generations (left) and the observed copy numbers of the bw^{75} allele in populations of D. melanogaster kept at sixteen individuals per generation (Buri 1956, right).

```
> par(mfrow=c(1,2))
```

Looking at the two plots (Fig. 6.5), we should see that the bw^{75} allele behaved very similarly to the binomial sampling model for our hypothetical A allele. By the end of both the simulation and the experiment, we see that the highest peaks are observed in the far left "Extinct" state (zero A/bw^{75} alleles) and the far right "Fixed" state (as many A/bw^{75} alleles as there are loci). This suggests that without any other forces acting on individual alleles, over time every new variant will either disappear or no longer be a noticeable variant, as it becomes the only allele at a site. The decay of the central peak over a wide range of probabilities should bring to mind diffusion of heat in physics (inspiring the "diffusion approximation" of the neutral theory); however, the absorbing boundaries at frequencies of zero and one are ultimately where the probabilities are concentrated.

So why should we be observing any level of genetic variation within populations? Mutation rates are certainly a factor, but we've already seen that new variants are quite likely to disappear almost as soon as they arise. So let's think about some reasons for seemingly neutral alleles to stick around in a population. We saw earlier (Fig. 6.4) that population size can influence the fixation and extinction probabilities of individual alleles. Let's visualize this effect again, but this time looking at multiple different simulations at once. We will use `rbinom` to randomly draw the number of alleles in each generation, based on the population size and their starting frequency:

```
> init_p <- 0.05 #Initial allele frequency

> gen <- 100 #Number of generations

> reps <- 10 #How many replicates to run
> colors <- rainbow(reps) #Grab some colors for our reps.

> N <- 10 #Set the population size

> #Initialize a plot that we can add lines to later
> plot(x=NULL, y=NULL, xlim=c(1, gen), ylim=c(0,1),
    xlab="Generations", ylab="Allele frequency")

> #For each replicate: draw new copy numbers of the allele
    per generation, then re-set the allele frequency 'p'
    and use that frequency for the next random draw
> for(i in 1:reps){
    p <- init_p
    for(j in 1:(gen-1)){
        a <- rbinom(n=1,size=2*N,prob=p[j])
        f <- a/(2*N)
        p <- c(p,f)
        }
    lines(x=1:gen, y=p, lwd=2, col=colors[i])
}
```

Try running the above code a few times with different population sizes (changing N from 10 to 100, for example). In Fig. 6.6, we show two examples from running the above code at different population sizes. You may notice that at smaller population sizes alleles seem to either go extinct or become fixed more frequently than in larger populations. And as a

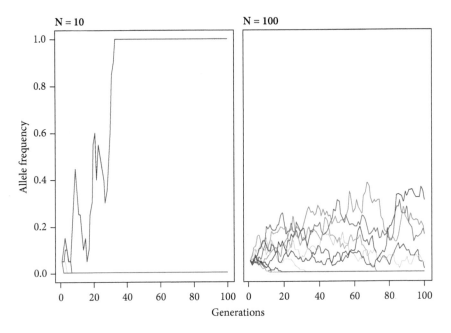

Figure 6.6 Ten replicates of random drift from a starting allele frequency of 0.05. A smaller population (left) loses all but one variant, but that one variant rises to become fixed in the population. A larger population loses half of its variants, and the remaining half stay fluctuating at moderate frequencies.

population gets larger, alleles seem to stick around for longer periods of time. However, try also changing the number of generations (Gen) in this simulation. Organisms can have radically different generation times: in the time between two salmon runs you might see ten, twenty, or more generations of fruit flies come and go. How do larger populations compare to smaller ones if you run them for 1,000 generations, as opposed to 100? Loss of variation over time is almost guaranteed, but factors such as population size and generation time significantly affect how rapidly we expect alleles to be lost in a population.

Finally, here is a simulation of genetic drift that keeps track of different trajectories and averages them when completed (Fig. 6.6). You can adjust starting frequencies and population sizes, and while the individual trajectories go all over the place, the average plotted at the end in the thick black line remains essentially unchanged (Fig. 6.7).

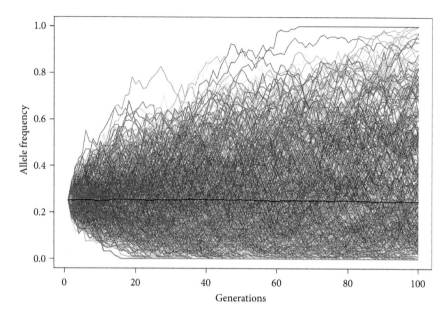

Figure 6.7 Five hundred replicates of random drift in a population of 100 individuals, starting with an allele frequency of 0.25. The average allele frequency across all replicates is plotted in black and stays close to the initial allele frequency.

```
> init_p <- 0.25 #Initial allele frequency
> gen <- 100 #Number of generations
> reps <- 500 #Lots of replicates to run
> colors <- rainbow(reps) #Grab some colors for our reps
> N <- 100 #Population size

> #Initialize a plot
> plot(x=NULL, y=NULL, xlim=c(1, gen), ylim=c(0,1),
    xlab="Generations", ylab="Allele frequency")

> Freq <- NULL #Create an object to save each replicates output

> #Iterate through the replicates
> for(i in 1:reps){
    p <- init_p
    for(j in 1:(gen-1)){
```

```
      a <- rbinom(n=1,size=2*N,prob=p[j])
      f <- a/(2*N)
      p <- c(p,f)
      }
   Freq <- rbind(Freq, p) #Save p
   lines(x=1:gen, y=p, lwd=2, col=colors[i])
}

> #Add the mean of all the replicates to the plot
> lines(1:gen, colMeans(Freq), lwd=2, col="black")
```

6.3 Quantifying variation

We've so far established that drift occurs relatively quickly in small populations, which can lead to the rapid loss of alleles over time. Take a look
at Veale et al. (2015) for a real-world example of dramatic genetic drift
in the stoat (*Mustela erminea*). To describe this loss of genetic variation
over time, Sewall Wright (Wright 1922) came up with a summary statistic
called the *fixation* index (*F*), which gave rise to a whole family of descriptive
F-statistics. We should point out here that the summary statistics that we'll
talk about in the rest of this book can be derived in multiple different
ways. For example, the fixation index can be derived by looking at the
percentage of heterozygotes, the rate of selfing in asexually reproducing
plants, or, as we'll see here below, the probability of two alleles descending
from the same copy of an allele in a pedigree. Don't be thrown when looking
through the literature and seeing multiple ways to calculate the same thing
(or the same symbols and similar words being used to describe different
things). Population geneticists are not the best at coming up with brand
new symbols for every new way to quantify phenomena.

   As we know, a diploid population of size N has $2N$ possible copies of
an allele. Assuming the population size is constant, what is the probability
that two randomly chosen alleles in one generation both originated from
the same copy of that allele in the generation before? For two alleles it

doesn't matter which allele we pick first, but for the second allele we pick to compare, we're interested in the probability that it comes from the exact same parental copy as our first allele. This constrains the possible origin of this second allele so it only has a $1/2N$ chance of coming from that same parental copy as the first allele. When two alleles have come from the exact same ancestral copy, we call them *identity-by-descent* or IBD. So our total probability that two random alleles sampled from a diploid population are the same is $F = \dfrac{1}{2N}$.

Conversely, the probability that two alleles were *not* from the same copy in the preceding generation is just $1 - F$ or $1 - \dfrac{1}{2N}$, which is a measure of genetic diversity often just called heterozygosity (H). If F is our per-generation probability of two alleles *not* being different, then H is just our per-generation probability of maintaining genetic diversity. We can use these values to define the rate of loss of heterozygosity in each generation by quantifying the expected relative change in heterozygosity from a starting value. If we know the starting amount of heterozygosity in generation g, H_g, then the remaining heterozygosity expected in the next generation is

$$H_{g+1} = H_g \left(1 - \frac{1}{2N}\right).$$

The process repeats itself in each generation, with every new generation's value of H modified by $1 - \dfrac{1}{2N}$, so we can jump forward in time g generations from an initial heterozygosity of H_0 like so:

$$H_g = H_0 \left(1 - \frac{1}{2N}\right)^g.$$

As we increase the number of generations we consider, $\left(1 - \dfrac{1}{2N}\right)^g$ actually converges on Euler's constant e, so we can switch from discrete time to a continuous time approximation:

$$H_g = H_0 \left(1 - \frac{1}{2N}\right)^g \approx H_0 \times e^{-g/2N}.$$

Let's visualize this process across some different population sizes:

```
> N <- c(10,50,100)
> gen <- 100
> het_init <- 1.0

> line <- c(1,2,4)
> colors <- c("orange", "black", "cyan")

> het <- sapply(1:gen ,function(x) het_init*exp(-(x/(2*N)))))

> plot(x=NULL, xlim=c(1,gen),ylim=c(0,1),
    xlab="Generations", ylab="Genetic diversity")

> for(i in 1:nrow(het)){
    lines(1:gen, het[i,], col=colors[i],
    lty= line[i], lwd=2)
}
> legend(x="bottomleft", legend=N, inset=c(0,1), xpd=TRUE,
    bty="n", col=colors, lty=line, lwd=2)
```

Starting with 100% of alleles being different, we see a slow and steady decay in diversity over time (Fig. 6.8). This reduction in genetic diversity over time is the generally assumed result of genetic drift, and the rate of loss is influenced by population size. The decay in heterozygosity is a non-equilibrium process. Without new variants being introduced by mutation or migration, we expect variation to eventually disappear. However, we do expect healthy populations to be able to exist at a "mutation-drift equilibrium," a point at which the population is large enough that it's not losing variants much faster than it can accumulate new ones. This equilibrium perspective is useful when thinking about a population that has become much smaller than it was previously, so that the variation that existed in the population at mutation-drift equilibrium can no longer be maintained.

One example is the Hawaiian crow or ʻalalā (*Corvus hawaiiensis*, See *Fig. 6.9*), which was extinct in the wild and maintained in captivity for decades as a population of approximately 100 individuals. What is the expected time for half of the genetic variation (defined as heterozygosity) averaged across the genome to be lost due to genetic drift under these

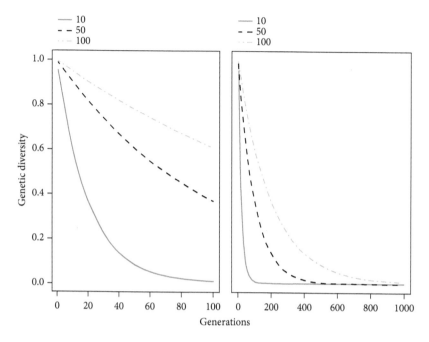

Figure 6.8 Rate of genetic diversity (*H*) loss in populations of different sizes, across two different time scales. Over longer time spans, large populations are expected to follow the same trend as smaller populations.

circumstances? To answer this, we can solve for *g*

$$H_g = H_0 e^{-g/(2 \times N)}$$
$$g = -(2N) \times \log_e(H_g/H_0)$$

then set $H_0 = 2$, $H_g = 1$ (or any ratio of 2:1), and calculate *g*.

```
> -2*100*log(1/2)
[1] 138.6294
```

So half of the original variation is expected to still exist after about 138 generations (at a constant population size of 100, with no selection, and with all individuals equally likely to reproduce).

Finally, the treatment of the change in *H* is a deterministic expectation (or average over a large number of loci); however, it should be clear from

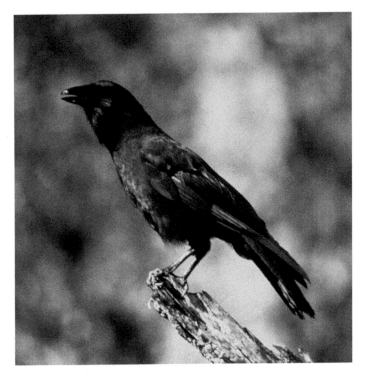

Figure 6.9 The Hawaiian crow or 'alalā (*Corvus hawaiiensis*). Photo from the US Fish and Wildlife Service.

the simulations that there is a large variance around the expected change in allele frequencies for a single locus. It is important to be aware of these two perspectives (single locus and genome average) simultaneously when thinking about and interpreting genetic drift.

The variance in allele frequency between generations due to drift is

$$\sigma^2 = \frac{p(1-p)}{2N}.$$

This makes some sense, since drift of two alleles is binomial and the variance expected from binomial sampling is

$$\sigma^2 = np(1-p).$$

However, it looks like the sample size, n or $2N$, is in the wrong place. This is because the variance is rescaled to be a proportion out of a total range of $2N$ with a caveat that variance is squared, which gives $4N^2$:

$$\sigma^2 = \frac{2Np(1-p)}{4N^2} = \frac{p(1-p)}{2N}.$$

6.4 Equilibrium heterozygosity and effective population size

Earlier we talked about the decay of heterozygosity in a small population with the ʻalalā example. However, we can also talk about expected heterozygosity at mutation-drift equilibrium: the rate of input of new mutations (2μ) is counterbalanced by the rate of removal of existing genetic variation by genetic drift (both forces are considered in terms of pairs of alleles):

$$2\mu(1-H) = H \times 1/(2N).$$

Note that if H is small, $1 - H \approx 1$:

$$H = 4N\mu.$$

Another derivation is given in the last chapter when discussing the coalescent.

However, predicted levels of genetic variation often do not match what is expected from actual "census" population sizes. This has led to the concept of an effective population size, N_e; in other words, the population size that would lead to observed levels of genetic diversity in an idealized (random mating, equal probability of reproducing, constant population numbers) population.

Humans are a perfect example of this distinction. The per-nucleotide, per-generation mutation rate has been estimated as on the order of 10^{-8} (for example, Tian et al. 2019). Average nucleotide heterozygosity—the rate at which a pair of DNA sequences differ in humans and would form a heterozygote if paired together in an individual—is on the order of one difference out of approximately 1,600 DNA base pairs or 0.0006 per base pair (for example, Stephens et al. 2001). Solving for N_e gives us $N_e = H/(4\mu)$, so given our measures of mutation rate and heterozygosity we can calculate the human N_e:

```
> H <- 0.0006
> u <- 10^-8
> H/(4*u)
[1] 15000
```

This should come as quite a shock. Our genetic diversity implies that there are only about 15,000 humans alive on the planet in any given generation! However, our census size is, at the time of writing, $N \approx 7.6 \times 10^9$; how can this be so far off?

There are a number of complexities to this, but to cut a long story short, one of the major factors is that genetic variation can quickly be lost but takes a long time (through slow mutations and genetic drift) to be regained.

To illustrate, let's have a population that switches between two sizes over time, N_1 for t_1 proportion of the time, and N_2 for the remaining t_2 part of time. Drift will be accelerated when it is at the smaller size and slow down at the larger size. How do we estimate an "effective" population of constant size that has the same overall rate of genetic drift as the oscillating population? One natural way to do this is to set the variance of the constant equal to the average variance (σ^2 from earlier) of the changing population:

$$\frac{p(1-p)}{2N_e} = t_1 \frac{p(1-p)}{2N_1} + t_2 \frac{p(1-p)}{2N_2}.$$

The first thing we can do is cancel out shared terms and simplify:

$$\frac{1}{N_e} = t_1 \frac{1}{N_1} + t_2 \frac{1}{N_2}$$

$$N_e = \frac{1}{t_1 \frac{1}{N_1} + t_2 \frac{1}{N_2}}.$$

This pattern, the reciprocal of the average reciprocals, is called the harmonic mean. The effective population size is expected to be equal to the harmonic mean of individual population sizes over time. Smaller numbers have larger effects on harmonic means. In population genetics, this means that accelerated drift in smaller populations can have a dominant lasting effect.

This is generalizable to an arbitrary number of population sizes and corresponding times:

$$N_e = \sum_i \left(\frac{t_i}{N_i}\right)^{-1}.$$

For our species, this means that we went through a bottleneck of less than 15,000 people in our past. Other human populations essentially went extinct (except for living on in small portions of our genome), and our numbers were dangerously low as well until we rebounded.

6.5 Overlapping generations

A final note is the issue of overlapping generations. Because of historical inertia, much of classical population genetics is based on discrete non-overlapping generations, known as a Wright–Fisher model (refer back to section 6.1), which is appropriate for annual plants or some types of invertebrates. However, many species are better modeled in continuous time as a range of ages at any given time where an individual death is replaced by an individual birth—known as a Moran model and popular in evolutionary game theory—rather than an entire generation at once. In reality, wild populations are somewhere in between these extremes; for example, even with overlapping generations individuals are more likely to reproduce in a particular age range. In general there is not much difference between essential results other than adjusting the rate of change. For example, the rate of genetic drift in a purely Moran model is twice the rate of drift in a purely Wright–Fisher model (the allele frequency changes within a generation instead of only between generations). However, if there is extreme unevenness, such as with plant seed reservoirs in the soil, "lost" alleles can be recaptured by germination of older seeds and the effective population size is increased. We've now focused a fair bit on random change in allele frequencies.

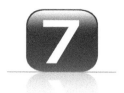

Adaptation and Natural Selection

7.1 Positive selection

Despite all our talk of neutral variation, early population genetics was mostly focused on questions of adaptation; specifically, the change in a species brought about by natural selection, such as differences in average survival and reproduction of individuals influenced by heritable genetic

Population Genetics with R: An Introduction for Life Scientists. Áki J. Láruson and Floyd A. Reed, Oxford University Press (2021). © Áki J. Láruson & Floyd A. Reed.
DOI: 10.1093/oso/9780198829539.003.0007

variation in the population. The myriad of forces that drive this process are generally referred to as the nebulous "natural selection."

There are many clear examples of "natural" selection which are associated with anthropogenic forces: pesticide resistance (Aminetzach et al. 2005), industrial melanism (van't Hof et al. 2011), herbicide resistance (Délye et al. 2013), and domestication (Purugganan and Fuller 2009). These are sometimes distinguished as "artificial" selection, but the boundary between the two can get quite murky. We'll generally just use the term "selection" to refer to non-neutral processes that drive changes in allele frequencies.

Some alleles may affect an organism's survival and reproduction; organisms carrying these alleles may be more likely to pass them on to the next generation. In these cases selection influences the change in allele frequencies over the generations because of differences in the resulting phenotypes. (An often unspoken assumption is that there is a genetic basis for these phenotypes; however, no matter how much variation exists, if it is not heritable and has a genetic basis, selection in an evolutionary sense is "blind" to it.) What is the predicted change in allele frequency when there are fitness differences conferred by selected alleles, and how can genetic variation be maintained in the face of selection? Answering these questions remains a major goal of population genetics today.

Let's start by considering selection acting only on individual alleles (that is, "haploid" or "genic" selection). This is a departure from our near-constant focus on diploids up to now, but don't worry: we'll broaden this out to diploid genotypes soon. Imagine that our allele *a* from our neutral drift simulation in Chapter 6 actually conferred some type of evolutionary advantage; maybe it increased the allosteric site affinity of a cell surface protein, resulting in more efficient oxygen transport and therefore greater survival odds when under physical duress, or maybe it allowed for a particularly sexy hair color. The exact nature of our selection force really doesn't matter; the only thing we're focusing on is that *something* is affecting the probability that this allele gets passed on down through the generations.

When we compare the two alleles A and a, we can think about their respective probabilities of being inherited. If both alleles have the exact same effects on fitness (that is, are selectively neutral to one another) the only thing that influences their probability of inheritance is their respective starting allele frequencies. But we're now saying that the A allele has an extra edge over a and has a fitness advantage of s (often referred to as a selection coefficient), so that its fitness relative to a is now $1 + s$, while the a allele has a fitness of 1.

If we think about the neutral fluctuation that happens in each generation, we can now add a step in each one where we adjust the probability of the allele being passed on (if it is first chosen randomly), based on its relative fitness:

$$P(\text{inherit A}) = \frac{1 + s}{2 + s}$$

$$P(\text{inherit a}) = \frac{1}{2 + s}.$$

We can see that if the selection coefficient is zero, then these both become 1/2, and we are back in the situation of neutral genetic drift.

The change in frequency of the A allele under genic selection in a subsequent generation must then be related to the product of its frequency (p) and relative fitness ($1 + s$). But we have to standardize that to include the effect of the a allele's relative fitness. If the frequency of a is then $1 - p$ and its relative fitness is 1, in our simple haploid selection example we can then calculate the change in allele frequency in the next generation ($t + 1$) as:

$$p_{(t+1)} = \frac{p(1 + s)}{p(1 + s) + (1 - p)(1)} = \frac{p(1 + s)}{ps + 1}.$$

Let's visualize this by simulating the process of a genic selective force influencing the variation of the a allele frequency over time. We can use our drift code from the last chapter and modify it slightly to incorporate a selection coefficient (*s*). First let's create a neutral reference point for ourselves:

```
> p <- 0.25 #Initial allele frequency

> gen <- 100 #Number of generations

> N <- 1000 #Population size

> #Initialize a plot that we can add lines to later
> plot(x=NULL, y=NULL, xlim=c(1,gen), ylim=c(0,1),
    xlab="Generations", ylab="Allele frequency")

> for(j in 1:(gen-1)){
    #Draw the number of alleles
    a <- rbinom(n=1,size=2*N,prob=p[j])
    f <- a/(2*N) #Get the allele frequency
    p <- c(p,f) #Save the frequency
}

> lines(x=1:gen, y=p, lwd=2)
```

You should see something similar, but not identical, to Fig. 7.1, where the allele frequency of *A* wanders up and down without clear direction over the generations. Under this scenario, the sampling of a particular allele only depends on its frequency in the population. Now let's explore the cases where it is not this simple and selection also influences the change in allele frequencies over time. We can easily modify the previous code to now consider the effect of selection and drift in each generation. To do this, we'll incorporate $p(1 + s)/(ps + 1)$ into our frequency calculation. Let's give our allele a 10% fitness advantage ($s = 0.1$), which should result in a rapid rise in frequency from 25% to 100% in less than 100 generations.

```
> p <- 0.25 #Initial allele frequency

> gen <- 100 #Number of generations
```

```
> N <- 1000 #Population size

> s <- 0.1 #Selection coefficient

> #Initialize a plot that we can add lines to later
> plot(x=NULL, y=NULL, xlim=c(1,gen), ylim=c(0,1),
    xlab="Generations", ylab="Allele frequency")

> for(j in 1:(gen-1)){
    #Draw the number of alleles
    a <- rbinom(n=1,size=2*N,prob=p[j])
    f <- a/(2*N) #Get the allele frequency
    #Modify the frequency by s
    p <- c(p,(f*(1+s))/(f*s+1))
}

> lines(x=1:gen, y=p, lwd=2)
```

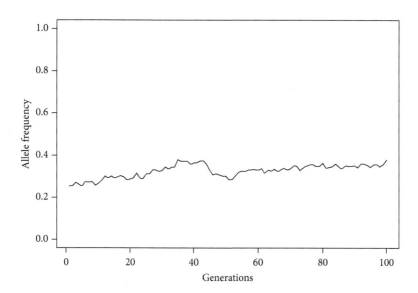

Figure 7.1 Changes in allele frequency over time influenced exclusively by genetic drift.

This time you should see something quite similar to Fig. 7.2. A 10% fitness advantage clearly has a significant effect on our allele frequency. In fact, it doesn't take much for genic selection to pretty drastically alter an allele's trajectory over time. Try increasing and decreasing the value of the selection coefficient, and re-run the code to see what affects the allele frequency over time. The selection coefficient can also have a negative value to represent an allele that's deleterious to an individual's fitness. In Fig. 7.3 we've chosen just five example values of s to highlight. Notice that when the selection coefficient is equal to zero, we only have genetic drift affecting the cross-generational fluctuations in allele frequency (that is, selective neutrality).

We've been running these simulations with a pretty large population size. We saw in Chapter 6 that population size can affect the probability that an allele drifts toward fixation or extinction. Specifically, we saw that in smaller populations an allele is more likely to drift toward fixation or extinction, rather than persisting in a population at intermediate

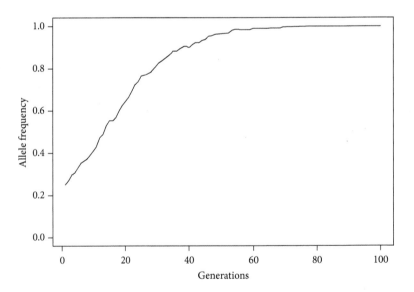

Figure 7.2 Changes in allele frequency over time influenced by both genetic drift and selection ($s = 0.1$).

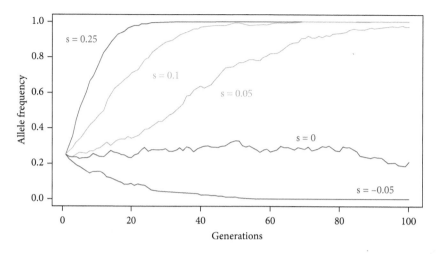

Figure 7.3 Select examples of drift and selection influencing allele frequency over time ($N = 1{,}000$) with different magnitudes of the selection coefficient.

frequencies. So what role does population size play now that we have both drift and selection operating simultaneously? When $s = 0$ (that is, when we have only neutral drift influencing our allele trajectories through the generations) the effects of this large population size should be apparent in how our allele frequencies most often seem to sway around our starting allele frequency, only rarely dropping much lower or ascending much higher. In this large population ($N = 1{,}000$), a 5% selection coefficient will reliably bring our allele up to near fixation in most of our runs. Let's see what happens when we drop our population size precipitously and run our code with our 5% selection coefficient:

```
> N <- 10 #A much smaller population size

> s <- 0.05 #Selection coefficient
```

The stark effects of population size should be readily apparent. Suddenly fixation and extinction are effectively random, despite the allele's selective advantage. In Fig. 7.4, we see results for the same five levels of our selection coefficient that we showed in Fig. 7.3, but with our much smaller population size of $N = 10$. Clearly the effects of selection can

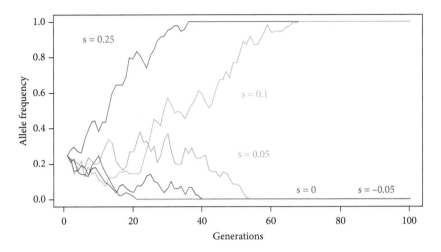

Figure 7.4 Examples of drift and selection influencing allele frequency over time with a much smaller population ($N = 10$).

be somewhat derailed by the force of genetic drift when a population is small. In fact, if you run this simulation multiple times, you'll see that even high selection coefficients can fail at maintaining our allele in the population at small population sizes. This is the phenomenon of how the forces of drift and selection can shift depending on the size of the population under consideration. A larger population should generally be able to hold onto variants that are neutral or under moderate selection over time, and strongly positively selected alleles can be expected to reach fixation relatively quickly. A small population, on the other hand, could be just as likely to have a neutral allele fix as a moderately positively selected allele. Even strongly selected alleles in a small population might not reach fixation quickly and might even be lost despite their advantage. This issue feeds into much of the focus of conservation genetics, since a major concern for endangered wild populations is that reduced population numbers mean that randomness is more of a contributor to future genetic make up than adaptive forces.

7.2 Adaptation, diploidy and dominance

The classical perspective of molecular adaptation is one of positive selection. For a new mutation to matter in an evolutionary sense, it has to increase by selection when rare. The lowest selection coefficient in the last examples was negative, so the allele had a relative fitness loss and was usually removed from the population pretty quickly. This type of selection is referred to as negative or purifying selection, and while it may seem trivial at first (rare mutations that are quickly lost will have little general or long-term effect on the population) it is a very important category of selection. We'll re-visit negative selection just a little later.

For now, let's tackle the question of selection on diploids. All our examples of selection earlier were of genic selection: selection acting only on individual alleles. But with two alleles a diploid produces three possible genotypes (*AA, Aa, aa*), and each genotype can have a fitness advantage or disadvantage based on their own selection coefficients: s_{AA}, s_{Aa}, and s_{aa}. Let's use $w = 1 + s$ to symbolize the relative fitness of these three genotypes: w_{AA}, w_{Aa}, and w_{aa}.

Because we're dealing with genotypes, we can predict the frequency of just the *A* allele in the next generation ($p_{(t+1)}$) by multiplying the expected genotype frequencies (according to the Hardy–Weinberg equation) by their fitnesses. We do have to keep in mind that heterozygotes only contribute half of their frequency to the allele we're interested in, so we'll need to divide our expected heterozygote frequency, $2p(1 - p)$, in half to get $p(1 - p)$:

$$p_{(t+1)} = \frac{w_{AA} \times p^2 + w_{Aa} \times p(1 - p)}{w_{AA} \times p^2 + w_{Aa} \times 2p(1 - p) + w_{aa} \times (1 - p)^2}.$$

So the expected contribution of the *A* allele to the next generation from *AA* homozygotes is the frequency of these homozygotes, p^2, times their fitness, w_{AA}. The contribution from heterozygotes is only half of their frequency times their fitness, because they are only half made up of *A* alleles, and to keep the frequency in the next generation a fraction between zero and one, this is divided by the total contribution of all genotypes.

Now we can introduce the complexities of dominance. We briefly touched on this concept earlier when we discussed blood types; specifically, when the *A* and *B* alleles are paired with the *i* allele in heterozygotes, they still confer the A and B blood types, respectively. So we could say that the *A* and *B* alleles are dominant to the *i* allele and the *i* allele is recessive to both the *A* and *B* alleles. Just like with phenotypes, we can think of fitness effects as being dominant and recessive to each other. Let's say there is a fitness advantage of 10% associated with the *A* allele. Our homozygote fitness values are then pretty straightforward: $w_{AA} = 1.1$ and $w_{aa} = 1$. If the fitness advantage of the *A* allele is dominant, our heterozygote fitness will be the same as that of the *AA* homozygote: $w_{Aa} = 1.1$; if it is recessive, it will be the same as the *aa* homozygote: $w_{Aa} = 1$. However, dominance/recessive relationships are not necessarily so clean cut. You might observe a phenomenon called incomplete dominance, where the heterozygote has an intermediate fitness between the two homozygotes. In the case of incomplete dominance, where the heterozygote fitness is an exact average between the two homozygote genotype fitnesses, we'll use the term semidominance. These degrees of dominance predict different evolutionary trajectories. Let's run some short simulations to illustrate the effects of different types of dominance.

Before we get started on that, however, a quick comment on a new R object class we're going to be using. So far we've only been dealing with vectors, data frames, and matrices. Now we're adding "list" to our list of R classes. Lists are great for storing multi-tiered information. For example, if you want to store matrices, vectors, and data frames all together as a single object that still allows access to each one individually, throw them all together in a list!

```
> cool <- list(c(1,2,3), c("ABAC"), matrix(c(1,2,3)),
    data.frame(x=1:3,y=1:3))
> str(cool)
```

```
List of 4
 $ : num [1:3] 1 2 3
 $ : chr "ABAC"
 $ : num [1:3, 1] 1 2 3
 $ :'data.frame':   3 obs. of  2 variables:
  ..$ x: int [1:3] 1 2 3
  ..$ y: int [1:3] 1 2 3
```

To access individual elements within the list, you can use double brackets to call them, and then you can access elements within that element by using nested brackets, like so:

```
> cool[[1]] #The first element in our list
[1] 1 2 3

> cool[[1]][3] #The third element of that first element
[1] 3

> #Our fourth element is a data frame
> cool[[4]][1] #Its first element is the first column
  x
1 1
2 2
3 3

> #We can even use the standard [row,column] subset approach
> cool[[4]][1,]
  x y
1 1 1
```

Amazing. Now that we know our way around lists, let's put them to use. We'll start by specifying all the vectors that we're going to need. We're going to generate allele frequency projections for all three fitness scenarios (recessive, dominant, and semidominant) with the same code, so let's make a list containing our w_{AA} and w_{Aa} values for each one, as well as a matrix for our three starting allele frequencies.

Notice that we're assuming that w_{aa} is equal to one for all scenarios, so we're excluding it from our calculations.

```
> #Set a lower allele frequency than we used in our
    genic selection example earlier
> init_p <- 0.05

> gen <- 400 #How many generations to run

> #Each fitness scenario is set up to have the homozygous
    fitness first, followed by the heterozygous fitness
> rec <- c(1.1, 1) #Recessive fitness values

> dom <- c(1.1, 1.1) #Dominant fitness values

> sem <- c(1.1, 1.05) #Semidominant fitness values

> #Matrix carrying our frequencies for each fitness scenario
> p <- matrix(c(init_p,init_p,init_p))

> #Combine our three fitness scenario vectors into a list
> w <- list(rec, dom, sem)
```

Now that we've got our list of genotype fitness scenarios, let's write a function to calculate our projected allele frequency $p_{(t+1)}$. That way we can more easily repeat our calculation multiple times for each element in our list. We're going to write this function with a single list element in mind. So, instead of assuming that our input is a full list, we're going to write this function so that it can handle a single element within our list. If that seems confusing right now, don't worry! It will hopefully become more clear as we go.

```
> #Our function will take a list element X (fitness value)
    and an element p (allele frequency)
> FitFreq <- function(X, p){
    w_total <- X[1]*p^2 + X[2]*2*p*(1-p) + (1-p)^2
    p_t <- (X[1]*p^2 + X[2]*p*(1-p)) / w_total
    return(p_t)
}
```

Our function `FitFreq` should now be able to take in a list element and an allele frequency value, calculate the total fitness contribution of all genotypes (`w_total`), then use that value to standardize the individual fitness contributions of just the homozygous (`X[1]`) and heterozygous (`X[2]`) genotypes. The projected allele frequency $p_{(t+1)}$ will then be the output from this function (`return(p_t)`).

We can spot check this function to make sure it's working by feeding it individual elements from our fitness list and allele frequency matrix:

```
> FitFreq(w[[1]], p[[1]])
[1] 0.05023744
```

That seems to be working. Alright, now we can use another member of the `apply` family of functions (we used `sapply` back in section 5.2 to square individual elements of a data frame) to apply our function to the elements in our list. This time we're going to use the function `lapply` to iterate across the elements in our list and apply our function. We're then going to save the calculations from all three fitness scenarios by binding those values to our p matrix. We want to repeat this calculation across multiple generations so we can actually place everything into a generational `for` loop. Since we've already got our first generation values in p, we'll run from generation one (`1`) to one-minus the total number of generations (`gen-1`) to get values across our whole 400-generation range. Also, because we're expanding our p as we run, we're specifying within `lapply` that the value of p we're using is always going to be the last column of that matrix (`p[,ncol(p)]`):

```
> for(i in 1:(gen-1)){
    p <- cbind(p, lapply(seq_along(w),
        function(j, y, n) {FitFreq(y[[j]], n[[j]])},
        y=w, n=p[,ncol(p)]))
}
```

Notice that within `lapply`, the first command we give is `seq_along(w)`. What this does is create a sequence based on the number of elements in our list. We can then tell `lapply` that we're going to be applying a function and that we need to consider three elements to successfully run it (`j`, `y`, and `n`). We define `y` as our fitness list w, and `n` as the last column of our p matrix (`p[,ncol(p)]`). Because we don't define `j`, `lapply` understands that those are the values from our `seq_along` entry, which is a numerical sequence going from one to three. That's a fair bit to unpack, but now let's reap the rewards by plotting each row of our allele frequency matrix, p. We'll start with an empty canvas that we'll set up with `plot(x = NULL, ...`, specify some colors and line types to use, and then use `lines` to get the allele frequency projections for each one of the fitness scenarios. Finally, let's include a nice legend so we know which line is which:

```
> plot(x=NULL, xlab="Generations", ylab="Allele frequency",
    xlim=c(1,gen), ylim=c(0, 1))

> colors <- c("orange", "darkgreen", "cyan")
> line <- c(1,2,4)

> for(i in 1:nrow(p)){
    lines(1:gen, p[i,], lwd=2, lty=line[i], col=colors[i])
}
> legend("bottomleft",
    legend=c("Recessive","Dominant","Semi-dominant"),
    inset=c(0,1), xpd=TRUE, bty="n",
    col=colors, lty = line, lwd=2)
```

The fruit of all our labors should look similar to Fig. 7.5. We can see that dominant fitness effects have a faster initial rise in frequency when rare, but are slow to fix at high frequencies; recessive fitness effects are the opposite, barely increasing in frequency for a long time, before quickly rising to fixation. Semidominant fitness effects appear to be the most efficient diploid configuration in terms of the overall time until fixation. However, genic selection directly upon haploid genotypes remains the most efficient form of selection. Try re-running the genic selection code from earlier, starting with a 5% allele frequency and running for 400 generations. The allele

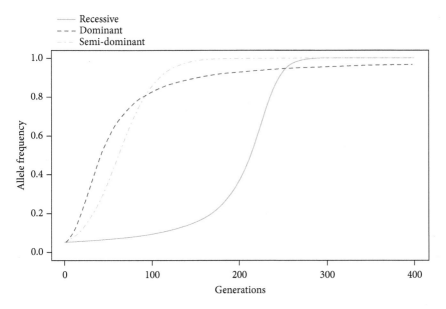

Figure 7.5 Projected allele frequency trajectories under recessive, dominant, and semidominant genotype fitness scenarios.

under genic selection should be reaching fixation at around generation 100, well before any other fitness scenario shown in Fig. 7.5.

If the fitness effect is semidominant, the predicted change in allele frequency can be linearized by a logit transformation (which is taking the natural log of your odds). Other types of dominance are nearly linear when transformed by a logit over a wide range of frequencies:

$$\ln\left(\frac{p}{1-p}\right) = y.$$

This allows us to estimate the selection coefficient from allele frequency data using a linear regression. To illustrate, let's look at real temporal allele frequency measurements from Fisher and Ford (1947) that show changes in allele frequency over eight generations in the scarlet tiger moth (*Callimorpha dominula*).

The allele in question (which appeared quite common at 89–90% frequency) affects the moth's wing pigmentation and could potentially be

Table 7.1 Temporal allele frequency shifts in scarlet tiger moths (*Callimorpha dominula*) from Fisher and Ford 1947.

Year	p
1939	0.908
1940	0.889
1941	0.932
1942	0.946
1943	0.944
1944	0.955
1945	0.935
1946	0.957

affecting survival due to predation (the wrong color pattern might give you away if you're trying to blend in), or mate preference and reproductive success (certain color patterns are more attractive than others), or any other selection story you can think up. In Fig. 7.6, we can see that the wings of the common homozygotes are red and black with yellow spots, while the rarer homozygotes (those without a copy of our measured allele) have way less spotting and generally darker wings. In addition, we can actually see that our measured allele is incompletely dominant, so that heterozygotes

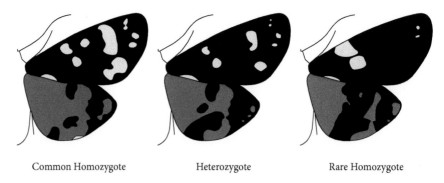

Common Homozygote   Heterozygote   Rare Homozygote

Figure 7.6 Phenotype examples of the scarlet tiger moth *Callimorpha dominula*, corresponding to three genotypes at a single locus. Note, however, that there is considerable individual variation of these general forms, illustrated after Clark et al. (1991).

are distinguishable from both homozygotes by having an intermediate phenotype.

Let's read in our moth dataset (this one is small enough that you can also type it in by hand if you want to) and run a linear regression with the `lm` function.

```
> data(moth) #Load the moth data set

> #Pull out the columns for easy manipulation
> Years <- moth$Years
> Freq <- moth$p

> #Linerize the allele frequencies
> logit<-log(Freq/(1-Freq))

> plot(Years, logit) #Plot our linearized data over time

> #Perform a linear regression
> (linear <- lm(logit ~ Years))

Call:
lm(formula = logit ~ Years)

Coefficients:
(Intercept)          Years
  -226.0923          0.1178

> #Use our regression object to plot the best fit line
> abline(linear)
```

Looking at the resulting plot in Fig. 7.7, it's apparent the allele is increasing in frequency over time. The slope of the regression best fit line is actually assumed to be approximately equal to the difference in fitness between heterozygotes carrying one copy of the allele and homozygotes carrying two copies. In our output we see that the slope is approximately 0.12; this gives us an estimate for the selection coefficient for the heterozygotes ($s_{+-} \approx 0.12$), and if we assume semidominance we can then estimate our remaining genotype fitnesses as $w_{++} = 1.24$, $w_{+-} = 1.12$, and $w_{--} = 1$,

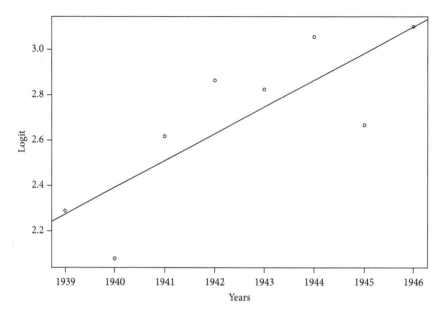

Figure 7.7 Linearized allele frequencies over time, from the scarlet tiger moth.

where "+" denotes the allele we're tracking in our data and "-" is the rarer allele that contributes to the darker phenotype. Note that we're using this approach to estimate a fitness value, but by itself this approach does not discriminate between natural selection and genetic drift. We're assuming that selection is the main driver of our allele frequency changes, but it's entirely possible that drift is playing a role. Also, the measurements are not independent from each other—the allele frequency of the following year depends on the frequency in the preceding year—which violates assumptions of many commonly used statistical tests (for more discussion of this see Waples 1989).

One very flexible framework for testing datasets is to generate simulated data under a model, in this case a null model of only genetic drift and no selection, and see where the observed results fall within the distribution of simulated results. Let's start by saving the squared correlation coefficient from our linear regression and use that as a key descriptor of our allele frequency changes over time:

```
> #Save our reference corr. coefficient for later
> (obs_r <- summary(linear)$r.squared )
[1] 0.6551432
```

So our observed data has an $r^2 \approx 0.655$. We can simulate thousands of datasets under a model of drift and count how frequently the simulated datasets exceed this r^2 value. We could even allow both our population size and the selection coefficient to vary to estimate the range of likely values for s_{+-}; however, that is a bit beyond the scope of this chapter.

Modifying the genetic drift code from Chapter 6, we can see just how often we could expect to see the same or greater value of r^2 if there was in fact no selection at all, and only drift was operating. Population size is going to play a big role here; we've already seen that as our population sizes get smaller, the effects of drift become much more pronounced and can easily drown out the effects of selection. So if we run this simulation with small population sizes, we're going to be amplifying the effects of drift. To guard against that, let's say that we're working with a population that's at least 1,000 individuals in size. That's not a humongous population, but it's large enough that we could reasonably assume that drift isn't drowning out all signatures of selection.

```
> #Start with the same frequency as the observed data
> initp <- 0.908

> #Set the same time frame as the observed data
> gen <- 8

> #Create a vector of our time frame for the regression model
> Years <- c(1:gen)

> #Let's replicate a neutral simulation 10,000 time
> reps <- 10000

> #Create a counting vector to keep track of our results
> count <- 0
```

```
> #Try a larger pop size to be more conservative
> N <- 1000

#A re-purposed drift loop
> for(i in 1:reps){
    p <- initp
    for(j in 1:(gen-1)){
        a <- rbinom(1,2*N,p[j])
        p <- c(p,a/(2*N))
    }
    logit <- log(p/(1-p)) #Linearize p
    reg <- lm(logit~Years) #Run a regression
    sim_r <- summary(reg)$r.squared #Get the r^2
    if(obs_r <= sim_r){ #Add 1 when r^2 exceeds threshold
        count=count+1
    }
}

#How often did we get the same or greater measure of r^2?
> count/reps
[1] 0.3349
```

From this we can see that the probability of seeing the observed data due to drift (as summarized by r^2, which is our stand-in for s_{+-}) is about 33%. That is high enough that we should reasonably be quite skeptical about any selection stories regarding this allele. As a final note on this dataset before we move on to other forms of selection, an earlier sample of scarlet tiger moths had an even higher frequency of the common allele. So at one point it was actually thought that selection was increasing the "-" allele frequency rather than decreasing it, as we see in the years from 1939 to 1946. This should underscore the caution that should be exercised when attempting to infer selection, because in addition to explaining the change by random drift, selection pressure (as well as population size) can fluctuate over time. Several studies have found evidence consistent with these kinds of fluctuations in insect populations over time.

Diploids are capable of even more fascinating examples of selection when the fitness of heterozygotes falls outside the range of the homozygotes. One form this can take is heterozygote advantage, or "overdominance," where the heterozygote is even more fit than either. The classic example of overdominance is the hemoglobin allele responsible for sickle cell anemia in humans in areas with a high incidence of malaria. In areas where malaria is rampant, heterozygotes have a fitness advantage due to increased malaria resistance in the altered red blood cells. However, homozygotes suffer from anemia and have an overall fitness cost despite malaria resistance. This appears to result in a stable equilibrium where the allele frequency is maintained at a certain level by selection. If it rises to a high enough frequency that more homozygotes are produced, the fitness cost results in fewer of those alleles being passed down. If it is at a lower frequency, heterozygotes are produced and the allele increases in frequency from an average fitness advantage. Let's look at data from Allison (1956) which collected hemoglobin genotype data for hemoglobin S from over 600 individuals in Tanzania.

Using the published genotypes, let's validate the observed and expected proportions under Hardy–Weinberg predictions:

```
> AA <- 400
> AS <- 249
> SS <- 5

> n <- AA + AS + SS
> print(paste("n:", n))
[1] "n: 654"

> p <- (SS + AS/2)/n
> print(paste("p:", p))
[1] "p: 0.198012232415902"

> EAA <- n*(1-p)^2
> EAS <- n*2*p*(1-p)
> ESS <- n*p^2
```

```
> print(paste("Observed:", AA/n, AS/n, SS/n))
[1] "Observed: 0.61162079... 0.38073394... 0.00764525..."

> print(paste("Expected:", EAA/n, EAS/n, ESS/n))
[1] "Expected: 0.64318437... 0.31760677... 0.03920884..."

> geno <- c(AA,AS,SS)
> expe <- c(EAA,EAS,ESS)

> G <- 2 * sum(geno * log(geno/expe))
> print(paste("G:",G))
[1] "G: 33.677475006339"

> pvalue <- pchisq(G, df=1, lower.tail=FALSE)
> print(paste("P-value:", pvalue))
[1] "P-value: 6.504958e-09"
```

Unlike the hemoglobin S data we saw in Chapter 5, these values deviate quite strongly from Hardy–Weinberg predictions, based on our likelihood ratio test. Given what we know about the potential fitness advantage of heterozygosity, what magnitude of heterozygote fitness advantage would be expected to maintain this allele frequency?

We can readily calculate this equilibrium point by setting the average fitnesses of the allele equal to each other. Let s represent the sickle cell causing allele at a frequency of p and a represent the common hemoglobin allele with three genotype fitnesses: w_{ss}, w_{sa}, w_{aa}. The s allele will either be paired with itself at a frequency of p and have a fitness of w_{ss} or with a at a frequency of $1 - p$ with a fitness of w_{sa}. This gives an average allele fitness of

Table 7.2 Hemoglobin data collected from over 600 individuals in Tanzania. From Allison (1956).

Genotype	AA	AS	SS	$\hat{p}$	Total
Individuals	400	249	5	0.199	654
Observed	0.612	0.381	0.008		
Predicted	0.643	0.318	0.039		

$$\bar{w}_s = w_{ss}p + w_{sa}(1 - p).$$

Using the same logic, the fitness of the *a* allele is

$$\bar{w}_a = w_{sa}p + w_{aa}(1 - p).$$

At equilibrium, $\hat{p}$, the average fitnesses are equal to each other:

$$\bar{w}_s = \bar{w}_a$$
$$w_{ss}\hat{p} + w_{sa}(1 - \hat{p}) = w_{sa}\hat{p} + w_{aa}(1 - \hat{p}).$$

Rearranging this to isolate the allele frequency gives

$$\hat{p} = \frac{w_{aa} - w_{sa}}{w_{ss} - 2w_{sa} + w_{aa}},$$

and rearranging for the heterozygote fitness gives

$$w_{sa} = \frac{\hat{p}(w_{ss} + w_{aa}) - w_{aa}}{2\hat{p} - 1}.$$

Allison (1956) estimated a threshold value for w_{ss} to be 0.2 in Musoma, Tanzania. If we set the relative fitness of $w_{aa} = 1$ and assume that the observed allele frequency is at equilibrium ($\hat{p} = 0.199$), we can calculate the assumed heterozygote fitness:

```
> p #Use the same allele frequency from earlier
[1] 0.1980122

> #Set the homozygote fitnesses
> w_ss <- 0.2
> w_aa <- 1

> #Calculate the expected heterozygote fitness
> (w_sa <- (p*(w_ss+w_aa)-w_aa) / (2*p-1))
[1] 1.262278
```

So what would we expect to happen if malaria could effectively be eradicated? Using our estimate of the fitness advantage conferred by being malaria resistant as a heterozygote, even in the face of significant health costs when the allele pairs up in homozygotes, let's look at the effects of multiple starting allele frequencies for the s allele. Then let's see what would happen if we were to remove the pressure imposed by the disease. We can repurpose the `FitFreq` function we wrote earlier:

```
> #Save our starting allele frequency from earlier
> init_p <- p

> #Save our two homozygous fitness values
> w_ss <- 0.2
> w_aa <- 1

> #Use the calculated heterozygous fitness value from earlier
> w_sa
[1] 1.262278

> #Start with 50 generations
> gen <- 50

> #Save our fitnesses as a single element in a list
> w <- list(c(w_ss,w_sa))

> #Let's try a range of different starting allele frequencies
> p <- matrix(c(0.01, 0.1, 0.2, 0.5, 0.9))

> #Save the sequence range of our starting frequencies
> iter <- seq_along(p)

> #Modify the lapply loop from earlier to use 'iter' as
    the first input and to only look at the one dominance
    scenario with y[[1]]
> for(i in 1:(gen-1)){
    p <- cbind(p, lapply(iter,
        function(i, y, n) {FitFreq(y[[1]], n[[i]])},
        y=w, n=p[,ncol(p)]))
```

```
}


> #Start a plot
> plot(x=NULL, xlab="Generations", ylab="Allele frequency",
    xlim=c(1,2*gen), ylim=c(0, 1))


> #Draw our results for the first 50 generations
> for(i in 1:nrow(p)){
    lines(1:gen, p[i,], lwd=2, col="blue")
}


> #Now let's take away the fitness scenario imposed by malaria
> w <- list(c(w_ss,1))


> #Start at our equilibrium frequency
> p <- matrix(init_p)


> #Update our iteration object
> iter <- seq_along(p)


> #Re-run our lapply loop for 51 generations
> for(i in 1:gen){
    p <- cbind(p, lapply(iter,
        function(i, y, n) {FitFreq(y[[1]], n[[i]])},
        y=w, n=p[,ncol(p)]))
}


> #Plot our lines from generation 50 to generation 100
> for(i in 1:nrow(p)){
    lines(gen:(2*gen), p[i,], lwd=2, col="red")
}
```

From the resulting plot (Fig. 7.8) we can see that if the fitness advantage is lost (that is, if malaria is largely eradicated) and the heterozygotes are equal in fitness to the common homozygote (ignoring anemia effects among heterozygotes), the s allele is predicted to drop to about a tenth (1/10) of its equilibrium frequency, from 0.2 to ≈0.02 over another fifty generations, and the rate of SS homozygotes suffering from anemia would drop two orders of magnitude from 4% (1 out of 25) to 0.04% (1 out of 2,500).

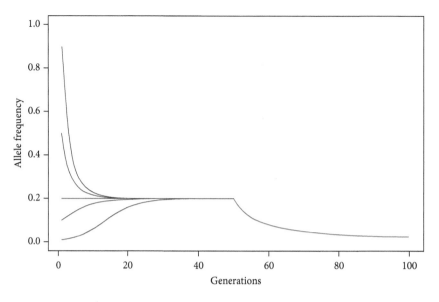

Figure 7.8 Allele frequency of the rarer allele over time from a range of starting points. Regardless of the starting allele frequency (and in the absence of drift), strong heterozygote advantage quickly leads to near-equilibrium allele frequencies. (This example is made to match the sickle cell anemia example given before: $w_{AA} = 1$, $w_{AS} = 1.27$, $w_{SS} = 0.2$.) For illustration, the heterozygote advantage is removed at generation 50 ($w_{AS} = 1$), which causes the allele frequency of S to drop rapidly.

The opposite of heterozygote advantage is underdominance, where the heterozygote has less fitness than either homozygote. A common form of this is found in chromosomal rearrangements such as reciprocal translocations, where two nonhomologous chromosomes exchange fragments (See Fig. 7.9). Half of the gametes from an individual that is a double heterozygote for a balanced translocation are imbalanced and after fertilization result in deleterious gene dosage effects from segmental aneuploidy. A useful approximation is that heterozygotes have half the fitness of homozygotes to model the dynamics. Of course, it is more complicated than this. This simplification assumes segmental aneuploidy is lethal, which may not always be the case. Taking into account mating between heterozygotes results in an even lower average fitness; a 3/8 fraction is viable. And some

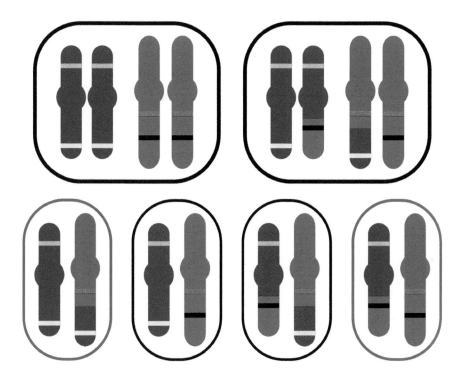

Figure 7.9 Top left: The normal diploid set of two chromosomes in a cell. The positions of genes on the chromosomes are indicated by color bars. Top right: A reciprocal translocation that has switched some genes between two of the chromosome copies. Lower: Four types of gametes that are produced in equal numbers from an individual with a reciprocal translocation. Half of these have duplicated and missing genes within the translocation (indicated in red); however, genes outside of the translocation are in their expected haploid copy number.

species have strong density-dependent effects where a lower fecundity does not directly translate into a proportional reduction in fitness.

The underdominance equilibrium can be calculated using the same formula, and logic, as the case of overdominance:

$$\hat{p} = \frac{w_{aa} - w_{sa}}{w_{ss} - 2w_{sa} + w_{aa}}.$$

Let's assume an underdominance case using the same code again. If we set $w_{ss} = 0.9$ and $w_{sa} = 0.5$, we have an underdominant scenario where the heterozygote is about half as fit as either homozygote (remember that we assume that $w_{aa} = 1$). First let's calculate what our equilibrium allele frequency would be:

```
> w_ss <- 0.9
> w_sa <- 0.5

> (p_eq <- (1 - w_sa)/(w_ss-2*w_sa + 1))
[1] 0.5555556
```

If our equilibrium allele frequency is just over 50%, let's see what allele frequency trajectories we could expect from starting allele frequencies ranging from 0.1 to 0.9:

```
> gen <- 20

> w <- list(c(w_ss,w_sa))

> p <- matrix(seq(0.1,0.9,0.1))

> iter <- seq_along(p)

> for(i in 1:(gen-1)){
    p <- cbind(p, lapply(iter,
        function(i, y, n) {FitFreq(y[[1]], n[[i]])},
        y=w, n=p[,ncol(p)]))
}

> plot(x=NULL, xlab="Generations", ylab="Allele frequency",
    xlim=c(1,gen), ylim=c(0, 1))

> for(i in 1:nrow(p)){
    lines(1:gen, p[i,],  lwd=2,  col="blue")
}

> p <- matrix(p_eq)
> for(i in 1:(gen-1)){
    p <- cbind(p, lapply(1,
        function(i, y, n) {FitFreq(y[[1]], n[[i]])},
```

```
        y=w, n=p[,ncol(p)]))
}

> lines(1:gen, p, lwd=2, lty="dashed", col="blue")
```

We can see from this (Fig. 7.10) that starting allele frequencies below our equilibrium frequency drop toward extinction pretty quickly, while those that start off just above are expected to increase to near fixation before too long. Unlike with overdominance, the underdominance equilibrium is not stable, and allele frequencies tend to move away from it rather than toward it. Because rare alleles are most often found as heterozygotes, underdominance translates into a rare allele disadvantage and the rare allele tends to be lost, even if the rarer homozygote is more fit than the alternative. Similarly, overdominance is best thought of as a rare allele

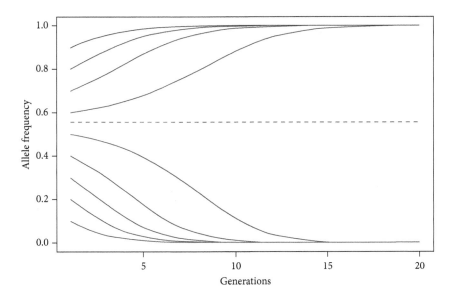

Figure 7.10 An example of the change in frequency, from a range of starting frequencies, with underdominance. In this example, the homozygote of the plotted allele frequency has a fitness of 90% and the heterozygote has a fitness of 50% relative to the remaining homozygote with a fitness of one. The (unstable) equilibrium is plotted with a dashed line.

advantage, since rare alleles tend to exist in heterozygotes, leading to a stable polymorphism. This illustrates one example of how evolutionary trajectories constrained by ploidy and fitness differentials can become trapped on less fit local fitness "peaks."

Early in population genetics it was speculated that widespread over-dominance may explain why so much genetic variation exists in a species (and that dominance itself evolves to fine-tune fitness). However, these hypotheses have largely fallen out of favor, and now a significant amount of genetic variation is thought to be selectively neutral.

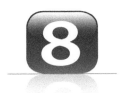

Population Differences

⊢ Term Definitions ⊢

Meta-population: An interconnected group of smaller populations.

Deme: A single population within a meta-population.

Sub-population: A group of individuals within a population that are more likely to breed with each other than members of other sub-populations.

8.1 Quantifying divergence

A common focus of population genetics is the quantification of differences between identifiable populations. One key measure of differences between populations that's been defined and redefined again and again (to consider different types of data, different assumptions of sampling approach, different numbers of other meta-population parameters, etc.) is F_{ST}. F_{ST} is one of the F-statistics derived by Sewall Wright (see Weir 2012 for additional information) and is broadly a quantification of the genetic differences between two related populations, generally ranging on a scale from zero (no difference) to one (complete difference). Conceptually, F_{ST} is a measure of how much of the total diversity is missing in different sub-populations, compared to the population at large.

Population Genetics with R: An Introduction for Life Scientists. Áki J. Láruson and Floyd A. Reed, Oxford University Press (2021). © Áki J. Láruson & Floyd A. Reed.
DOI: 10.1093/oso/9780198829539.003.0008

Based on Hardy–Weinberg expectations, we know the amount of diversity (that is, heterozygotes) we can expect when we have a measure of allele frequency is $2p(1 - p)$. If we have allele frequency measurements from multiple sub-populations, we can say that our total expected heterozygosity (H_T) is

$$H_T = 2\bar{p}(1 - \bar{p}),$$

where $\bar{p}$ is the average allele frequency across all the sub-populations. We can contrast this with the average of our observed levels of heterozygosity within each sub-population (H_S), which if we had two sub-populations would be

$$H_S = \frac{2p_1(1 - p_1) + 2p_2(1 - p_2)}{2} = \frac{H_1 + H_2}{2},$$

where p_1 is the allele frequency in sub-population 1 and p_2 the frequency from sub-population 2, and H_1 and H_2 are the respective measures of heterozygosity within each sub-population.

Let's visualize the relationship between H_T and H_S with the code below:

```
> #Let's choose two arbitrary allele frequencies to look at
> p1 <- 0.15
> p2 <- 0.7


> #Calculate the individual sub-pop measures of H
> h1 <- 2*p1*(1-p1)
> h2 <- 2*p2*(1-p2)


> #Calculate the average allele frequency
> p_ave <- (p1+p2)/2


> #Use average allele frequency to get total expected H
> ht <- 2*p_ave*(1-p_ave)


> #Use individual sub-pop H measures to get total observed H
> hs <- (h1 + h2)/2
```

```
> #Use the curve function to plot our expected H values
    across the full range of allele frequencies
> curve(2*x*(1-x), from=0, to=1, xlab="Allele frequency",
    ylab="Heterozygotes", lwd=2)

> #Plot our individual sub-pop values onto the curve
> points(c(p1,p2), c(h1,h2), cex=2, pch=16)

> #Plot our averaged values onto the curve
> points(c(p_ave,p_ave), c(hs,ht), cex=2)

> #Add some text to identify each point
> text(x=p1, y=h1-0.03, "H1")
> text(x=p2, y=h2-0.03, "H2")
> text(x=p_ave, y=hs-0.03, "HS")
> text(x=p_ave+0.03, y=ht-0.03, "HT")

> #Draw lines to connect the points
> lines(c(p1,p2), c(h1,h2), lty=2)
> lines(c(p_ave,p_ave), c(hs,ht))
```

From the plot we just made (Fig. 8.1), we can see that the $2p(1 - p)$ curve of expected heterozygosity is concave downward. Therefore, when populations have different allele frequencies with different expected heterozygosities (H_1 and H_2 in the figure) the combined midpoint between them (H_S on the dashed line) will always be lower than expected total heterozygosity (H_T).

The measure of F_{ST} is the fraction of "missing" heterozygosity between H_S and H_T, standardized by H_T:

$$F_{ST} = \frac{H_T - H_S}{H_T} = 1 - \frac{H_S}{H_T}.$$

The maximum amount any two measures of allele frequencies could differ is one being a 100% and the other being 0%. In that situation there are no heterozygotes, both our measures of H_1 and H_2 will be zero, and our $F_{ST} = 1 - (H_S/H_T) = 1 - (0/0.5) = 1$. If, on the other

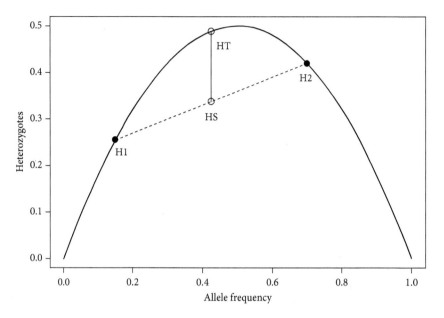

Figure 8.1 Relationship between expected total heterozygosity (H_T) and observed individual heterozygosity (H_S), with arbitrary allele frequencies from two sub-populations ($p_1 = 0.15, p_2 = 0.7$).

hand, our two measures of allele frequencies are identical between the two sub-populations, then both our measures of H_1 and H_2 will be the exact same, and any way we calculate the average we'll have the same value of $H_1 = H_2 = H_S = H_T$, (H_S/H_T) will equal 1, and $F_{ST} = 0$.

We can return to the human SNP data we plotted in Chapter 4 and take a closer look at observed and expected heterozygosity:

```
> data(snp)
> h_exp <- 2*snp$p*(1-snp$p) #Expected heterozygosity for
    #25 different alleles
> fst <- (h_exp-snp$het) / h_exp
> mean(fst)
[1] 0.09111416
```

Average F_{ST} across all loci works out to about 9% missing heterozygosity.

Is this a statistically significant level of F_{ST}? Like many things, there are a number of ways to test this. Some argue for using a multinomial likelihood framework that explicitly models F_{ST}; however, we can do two quick tests that are quite flexible for a range of circumstances. First of all, only one of the observed heterozygosities out of 25 is higher than its predicted value. If we assume that, by random chance, a calculated heterozygosity is equally likely to be higher or lower than its expected value, we can appeal to a binomial distribution and calculate that the probability of seeing this kind of deviation or greater is

$$25 \times (1/2)^{25} + (1/2)^{25} = 7.75 \times 10^{-7}.$$

We could also use a non-parametric test that makes no assumption about the underlying distribution of the data given the model, like the Wilcoxon signed-rank test,

```
> wilcox.test(h_exp, snp$het, exact = FALSE,
    paired = TRUE, alternative = "greater")
```

which gives a p-value of 9.421×10^{-6} (exact = FALSE is there to suppress an error from tied values).

Note that F_{ST} only quantifies differences between populations. It does not tell you, by itself, why the populations are different (for example, low rates of migration with drift, shared recent ancestry with isolation and drift, strong selection on a subset of loci that vary in fitness by location, etc.).

8.2 Relative likelihood of the population of origin

We can think of predicted genotype proportions as probabilities of seeing a certain set of alleles among individuals in a population. If populations differ in allele frequencies, we can use genotypes to infer relative likelihoods of an individual originating from each population.

Say we have a DNA sample from a blue whale (*Balaenoptera musculus*, See Fig. 8.2) sampled in the southern Pacific Ocean and we want to infer whether that individual originated from an Antarctic or Australian population (these are currently considered subspecies, *B. m. intermedia* and *B. m. brevicauda*). In Table 8.1, the actual genotypes of seven microsatellites from a blue whale.

Table 8.1 Genotypes at seven difference loci, sampled from a single blue whale.

Locus	Genotype
GATA28	189/201
GT023	135/145
Dde09	242/246
Bmy1	265/265
Bmy53	206/206
Bmy57	153/169
BM261	207/209

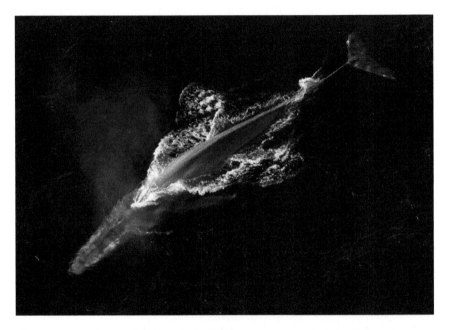

Figure 8.2 A photo of a blue whale (*Balaenoptera musculus*), the largest known animal. Photo from the US National Oceanographic and Atmospheric Administration.

We can use this table of whale genotypes to determine the frequencies of these alleles in the two whale populations (Attard et al. 2012). The dataset "whale" from our *popgenr* package contains a large number of whale genotypes from Antarctica and Australia.

```
> data(whale)
```

This dataset contains genotypes for 264 individual blue whales across seven distinct loci. Let's attempt to calculate the allele frequencies for each allele, specifically within each sub-population. To do this we'll need to count up each allele, first from one location, then the other. Because blue whales are diploid, each locus name has a subscript of either "_1" or "_2" to specify the two different copies of each locus. So we'll have to count up the alleles from two separate columns with two different names! We don't want to assume how the columns are arranged in the dataset; all we know is the naming scheme of the columns. So in order to do this, we'll use a very handy function called sub, a find and replace function which uses regular expressions (*regex*) to exactly match complex patterns. We can't properly go into all the details of *regex* here, but very briefly it is a way of succinctly describing very specific patterns, involving both text and formatting. For example, in our case we can use sub to remove everything in our column names up to and including an underscore, starting from the end of each name. We can accomplish this by simply using the regular expression _. and telling sub to replace all matches with nothing (" "). This is a very bare bones example, but we heartily encourage further familiarization with regular expressions, since their use is implemented in multiple programming languages and they are unmatched in terms of the speed and specificity with which they can search through and alter volumes of text. We'll also use a very handy function called table, which can quickly count up elements in a data frame or list:

```
> #Get all unique formatted locus names from the columns,
    omitting the first column which is ''Location''
> loci <- unique(sub(pattern="_.", replacement="",
    colnames(whale)[-1]))

> #Loop through each location, and within each
    location loop through all loci
> dat <- NULL
```

```
> for(i in unique(whale$Location)){
    x <- (whale[whale$Location==i,])
    for(j in loci){
        loc1 <- paste(j, "_1", sep="")
        loc2 <- paste(j, "_2", sep="")
        count <- table(c(x[,colnames(x)==loc1],
            x[,colnames(x)==loc2]))
        freq <- count/sum(count)
        y <- data.frame(i,j,freq)
        dat <- rbind(dat,y)
    }
}
> #Add column names to our new data frame
> colnames(dat) <- c("Location","Locus","Allele","Frequency")
```

Our resulting dataset should look something like this:

```
> head(dat)
    Location    Locus Allele   Frequency
1 Antarctica GATA028    165 0.106451613
2 Antarctica GATA028    169 0.032258065
3 Antarctica GATA028    177 0.003225806
4 Antarctica GATA028    185 0.054838710
5 Antarctica GATA028    189 0.183870968
6 Antarctica GATA028    193 0.229032258
```

The allele frequency information for our relevant alleles (that is, those that our mystery individual possesses) are summarized in Table 8.2.

Now that we have the per-population allele frequencies, we can use p_i^2 or $2p_ip_j$ to calculate our expected homozygotes and heterozygotes and then begin to get at the probabilities of the corresponding genotypes in our mystery whale occurring in either of the two populations:

$$P(x|\text{population}_i) = \prod_j \begin{cases} p_{k,i}^2, & \text{if homozygous} \\ 2p_{k,i}p_{l,i}, & \text{if heterozygous.} \end{cases}$$

Table 8.2 Selected blue whale allele frequencies from Antarctic and Australian population data in Attard et al. (2012). The values do not add up to one within a locus because there are additional alleles not shown.

Locus	Allele	Antarctica	Australia
GATA28	189	0.184	0.147
GATA28	201	0.155	0.344
GT023	135	0.0323	0.0184
GT023	145	0.152	0.197
Dde09	242	0.261	0.179
Dde09	246	0.232	0.564
Bmy1	265	0.281	0.550
Bmy53	206	0.310	0.872
Bmy57	153	0.090	0.596
Bmy57	169	0.106	0.0413
BM261	207	0.513	0.0642
BM261	209	0.190	0.624

The probability of the multilocus genotype data (x) from the ith population is the product of each genotype j which is a function of the corresponding allele frequencies (p_k or p_l) in population i, and is calculated according to zygosity of the genotype. We can now subset our data frame using multiple conditions and use the R terminal as a calculator to fill in Table 8.3:

```
> 2 * dat[dat$Location=="Antarctica" &
    dat$Locus=="GATA028" &
    dat$Allele==189,]$Frequency *
    dat[dat$Location=="Antarctica" &
    dat$Locus=="GATA028" &
    dat$Allele==201,]$Frequency
[1] 0.05694069

> 2 * dat[dat$Location=="Australia" &
    dat$Locus=="GATA028" &
    dat$Allele==189,]$Frequency *
    dat[dat$Location=="Australia" &
    dat$Locus=="GATA028" &
    dat$Allele==201,]$Frequency
[1] 0.1010016
```

```
> dat[dat$Location=="Antarctica" &
    dat$Locus=="Bmy1" &
    dat$Allele==265,]$Frequency^2
[1]  0.07876171

> dat[dat$Location=="Australia" &
    dat$Locus=="Bmy1" &
    dat$Allele==265,]$Frequency^2
[1]  0.3030048
```

Table 8.3 Whale genotype probabilities.

Locus	Genotype	Antarctica	Australia
GATA28	189/201	0.0569	0.101
GT023	135/145	0.00978	0.00723
Dde09	242/246	0.121	0.202
Bmy1	265/265	0.0788	0.303
Bmy53	206/206	0.959	0.760
Bmy57	153/169	0.0192	0.0492
BM261	207/209	0.195	0.0801

Assuming that the loci are independently inherited (that they are separated by sufficient recombination and not closely linked) we can multiply the individual genotype probabilities together:

```
> 0.0569 * 0.00978 * 0.121 * 0.0788
[1]  5.305945e-06
> .Last.value * 0.0959 * 0.0192 * 0.195
[1]  1.905097e-09
```

The example above gives us the overall probability of our mystery whale having come from the Antarctic population. Note the use of .Last.value to get the output of the line before in the next calculation. Multiplying across for both populations, we get pretty small probabilities that our blue whale came from either the Antarctic (1.905097×10^{-9}) or Australia (1.338643×10^{-7}). In fact, any individual compound genotype has a low probability of occurring, but we can compare the likelihood ratios of probabilities (the probability of the genotype in one population compared to the other),

$$\text{Ratio}_i = \frac{P(x|\text{population}_i)}{P(x|\text{population}_j)},$$

and the probabilities between the two populations out of the sum of both probabilities (the relative probability):

$$\text{Relative}_i = \frac{P(x|\text{population}_i)}{P(x|\text{population}_i) + P(x|\text{population}_j)}.$$

```
> (Ant <- 0.0569*0.00978*0.121*0.0788*0.0959*0.0192*0.195)
[1] 1.905097e-09
> (Aus <- 0.101*0.00723*0.202*0.303*0.760*0.0492*0.0801)
[1] 1.338643e-07

> (Rat_ant <- Ant/Aus)
[1] 0.01423155
> (Rat_aus <- Aus/Ant)
[1] 70.2664
> (Rel_ant <- Ant/(Ant+Aus))
[1] 0.01403186
> (Rel_aus <- Aus/(Ant+Aus))
[1] 0.9859681
```

These values are given in the "Ratio" and "Relative" columns of Table 8.4.

The relative probabilities are useful for visualizing the support for the two "models" of population origin. Let's visualize our results with a pie chart to mix things up a bit (See Fig. 8.3):

Table 8.4 Comparison of the two genotype probabilities.

Population	Π	Ratio	Relative
Antarctic	1.92×10^{-9}	0.0142	0.0140
Australia	1.34×10^{-7}	70.3	0.986

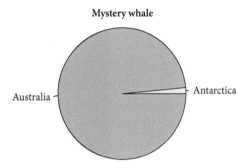

Figure 8.3 Relative population assignment of the whale sample based on multilocus genotypes.

```
> pops <- c("Antarctica", "Australia")
> color <- c("lightblue1","orange")
> slices <- c(Rel_ant, Rel_aus)

> pie(slices, labels=pops, main="Mystery whale", col=color)
```

Any single microsatellite is not diagnostic, and some of the genotypes are more likely in the Australian population, while others are more likely in Antarctica. However, with sufficient data, in this case seven microsatellites, we can build a stronger case for where our mystery whale likely originated. Our sampled whale is ≈70 times more likely to have come from Australia, and indeed this is the case. The genotypes of a blue whale sampled from the Australian population by Attard et al. (2012) were used in this example. The ratios of probabilities of the data under two models (in this case our population of origin) is known as a Bayes factor in statistics, and is often used for model selection (Kass and Raftery 1995).

We sidestepped an issue that will quickly be encountered when working on these kinds of questions and data. When an allele is missing from one population sample, this leads to an inference of a frequency of zero in that population. Thus any genotype containing that allele also has a probability of zero. However, we cannot be reasonably confident that the allele is completely missing from the population based on a finite sample. This has been addressed in the literature in various ways. Today the standard approach is to use a uniform prior of allele frequencies, update this distribution with the observed sampled alleles, and then use a Beta or Dirichlet distribution (depending on the number of parameters) as the basis of probability calculations (that is, a Bayesian approach).

8.3 DNA fingerprinting

As can be seen in the last section, when a number of variable loci are combined, the probability of a specific set of multilocus genotypes can be very small. Even though the genotypes of our mystery whale were more likely to have occurred in Australia, the set of seven microsatellites had a probability of 1.34×10^{-7}, which is less than one out of seven million. The upper-range estimate of the global number of blue whales today is 25,000.[1] In principle, a set of a sufficient number of genotypes can be used to uniquely identify a single individual. Comparisons of genotypes can also be used to support or refute genetic relationships such as paternity. This has applications in forensics as well as biology (where an understanding of the mating systems and individual reproductive success of various species has been revolutionized). Ultimately DNA fingerprinting (or DNA "profiling," as it is now more commonly referred to) is a question of genotype and allele frequencies.

The Federal Bureau of Investigation of the United States maintains an online database of collected genotyped loci that's publicly available.[2] This includes thirteen core "CODIS" (Combined DNA Index System) loci that have been adopted as a common standard for identification in the US. A subset of this data, genotyped in 1,036 people, can be loaded into R from the *popgenr* package.

```
> library(popgenr)
> data(thirteen)
```

[1] http://www.iucnredlist.org/details/2477/0.
[2] https://strbase.nist.gov/fbicore.htm.

Try using R and this dataset to calculate the probability of a hypothetical multilocus genotype at all thirteen loci. How does this compare to the current world human population estimate?

DNA fingerprinting has received a lot of attention, and there are a range of relevant issues involved. There is no room to go into detail here, and much of the development surrounds methodological details such as the choice of markers, allele binning strategies, probability calculations (which can become complex; for example, Weir 1992; Graham et al. 2000; Waits et al. 2001), etc. Interested readers are recommended to read Roewer (2013) and/or Chambers et al. (2014) for more details and a history of the field and its wide-ranging impacts. However, we do wish to highlight a few issues:

- Individuals are not random draws from a population but exist as clusters of relatives who are more likely to share genotypes with each other.
- Some individuals (identical monozygotic twins in humans, vegetative clones, or parthenogenic species) are essentially genetically identical. Detecting the rarer mutational differences among twins and taking into account somatic mutations would take a much more massive genotyping effort than is usually done.
- The selection of the appropriate reference population(s) to establish allele frequencies affects the calculation, and it is not always clear which population is the most appropriate reference. There are also ethical and legal issues associated with collecting genetic data from individuals (for example, Maryland versus King 569 US).
- Mutations do happen. Highly variable markers such as microsatellites are highly variable because they have a high mutation rate. Occasionally new mutations are seen and can complicate inference such as paternity analysis.
- Many of the concerns listed here make standard probability calculations less conservative; however, in general a sufficient number of markers will result in overwhelming probabilities that can overcome these issues.

- When critically interpreting DNA fingerprinting data, one must also consider nongenetic factors such as the possibility of contaminated or mixed samples, human errors (or purposeful forgery) like sample mislabeling, etc. These factors can have much higher probabilities than a genuine multilocus genotype match by random chance. See Anonymous (2009) for a possible example linking forty crime scenes over fifteen years.

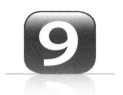

Pointing the Way to Additional Topics

Learning is always a lifelong endeavor; what we've covered in this book barely scratches the surface of all the complexities and nuances of drawing evolutionary inferences from genetic data. Learning is an iterative process and layers upon layers can be added to further refine your understanding. We have purposefully avoided some details for the sake of clarity and establishing a fundamental knowledge; for example, the way we calculated sample heterozygosities (as an estimate of heterozygosity in the population) in this book is slightly biased (refer to Nei and Roychoudhury 1974), but it can be difficult to understand why and in general does not greatly affect the calculations or interpretation—just know that what we cover here is not the end of the story, even for seemingly simple concepts. There is also not space to go into a range of important topics such as phylogenetics, quantitative genetics, Markov Chain Monte Carlo (MCMC) methods, Approximate Bayesian Computation (ABC), multiple testing issues, ascertainment bias, and similar additional topics.

Also, we haven't touched on some historical and social aspects of population genetics. Provine (1971) is highly recommended for people interested in a history of the development of population genetics. We would also be remiss if we didn't point out that many early population geneticists were also supportive of eugenics, and the history of eugenics programs is a topic

Population Genetics with R: An Introduction for Life Scientists. Áki J. Láruson and Floyd A. Reed, Oxford University Press (2021). © Áki J. Láruson & Floyd A. Reed.
DOI: 10.1093/oso/9780198829539.003.0009

about which there is a strong cultural amnesia in the US. Paul (1995) is recommended as a resource to begin learning about this history.

However, we hope that what we've provided will empower new and continuing students to explore and visualize data and models for themselves, to challenge models, build their own, and ask themselves what expectations are reasonable. Here is a non-exhaustive list of important additional population genetics topics (each could be developed into a book in its own right) that we will introduce to point the way to further understanding and exploration.

9.1 The coalescent

A very important concept in population genetics is focusing on the coalescence of lineages (lines of inheritance coming together) as we move backward in time over previous generations of a population. In this book we've almost exclusively dealt with "forward" simulations of genetic changes over time. However, modeling allele frequency changes backward through time is not only an interesting perspective when you know the current allele distribution within a population and you want to find out how it could have gotten to that point; computationally it can also be significantly faster than coding for random changes forward in time. To clarify this perspective, let's think some more about how inheritance works in a population. The simulation illustrated in Fig. 39 shows how alleles are randomly inherited from parents from the generations before in a small population. In the first generation all alleles are designated individually (which may or may not correspond to actual allele differences). Because in this simple model we do not have mutations, once an allele is lost by not being sampled by chance it cannot be gained again. Identity by descent (IBD, alleles originating from a single ancestral copy, introduced in Chapter 6) accumulates in each generation.

Importantly, we don't have to keep track of individuals. What is important here is keeping track of allele copies. This process of genetic drift is much easier to visualize when we sort the alleles by IBD.

As predicted, genetic diversity (heterozygosity values, in the sense of non-IBD, are listed on the right in Fig. 39) more or less declines until it reaches zero and all individuals contain alleles from a single initial copy (in this case it is copy #4). Note that allele copy #4 fixed in the population despite dropping to a single copy and was almost lost in generations 4, 10, and 11.

All alleles in the last generation are descended from the single copy in generation 11. However, the most recent common ancestor occurs later in generation 14, but this is difficult to see in this plot. In the next figure we'll indicate only the copies that are direct ancestors of the last generation.

Now something else should become clear that is not intuitive. Most alleles are *not* ancestors of later generations, even though most alleles do leave descendant copies in the immediately following generations. This is a surprising and general property of how genetic lines of inheritance work at a locus in a population. Compare the number of gray copies to the number of black copies in Fig. 40.

When modeling genetic drift, the last insight—that most alleles do not have descendants that ultimately matter (in a population-genetic sense)— implies that we don't have to keep track of an entire population. All we need to do is keep track of the lines of ancestry which come together to a common ancestor (this coming together of lineages is called *coalescence*). In fact, we don't have to keep track of all the individual steps along a lineage, we just need to know the distances in generations.

In this coalescent genealogy several common qualities are clear. The length between nodes (coalescent events) tends to be larger the deeper you go into the past. Conversely, there are many coalescent events in the last few generations. Most coalescents are bifurcations moving forward in time—a single lineage splitting into two lineages. However, in the last generation there are two trifurcations (split into three) and even one quadfurcation, which are often predicted in very small populations such as this.

Let's visualize the coalescence of two lineages. The process of coalescence can be approximated in continuous time by an exponential distribution with a rate parameter of $1/(2N)$ (the chance of coalescence in each

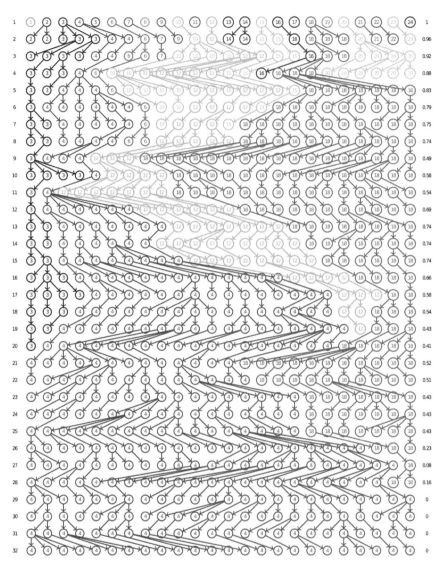

Figure 9.1 A coalescent process highlighting each ancestor variant's trajectory through time. Generations are listed on the left and heterozygosity on the right.

generation). We can write down an approximation for two lineages with the probability of coalescence at time t as

$$P(t) = \frac{e^{-t/(2N)}}{2N}.$$

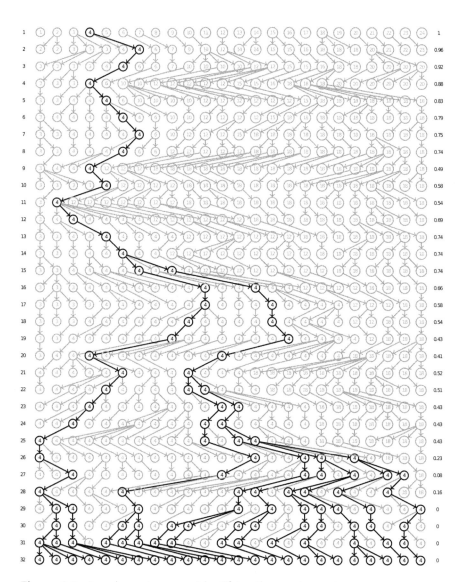

Figure 9.2 A coalescent process identifying the most recent common ancestor (MRCA) of all individuals in the last generation.

The mean of an exponential distribution is the inverse of the rate parameter $(1/(2N))^{-1} = 2N$ (keep in mind we are talking about $2N$ *generations* back in time—time in units of generations is scaled by the population size which affects the rate of coalescence in each generation because of the number of

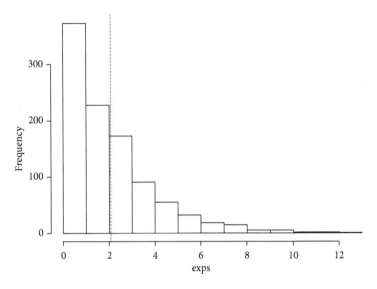

Figure 9.3 A thousand random draws from an exponential distribution, representing the distribution of coalescent events for pairs of lineages.

copies for lineages to choose from). We can model this in R by random draws from an exponential:

```
> exps <- (rexp(1000,1/2))
> hist(exps)
> abline(v=mean(exps), col='blue', lty=2)
```

This code generates 1,000 random draws from an exponential distribution with a rate of 1/2 (so the units are scaled in terms of N generations). It also calculates the average value and indicates it with a vertical dashed blue line; as expected, it is near $x = 2$.

We can add a predicted curve to the plot by adding this code:

```
> #Make a new vector of 1,000 evenly spaced points between
    0 and our maximum value
> q <- seq(0, max(exps),length = 1000)

> #Calculate the exponential density function for the q
    points with a rate = 1/2
> z <- dexp(q, 1/2)
```

```
> #Tell R to overlay the next plot
> par(new = TRUE)

> #Plot the fitted normal distribution over the histogram
    with the axes and axes labels removed
> plot(q, z, type = ''l", lwd = 1, axes = F, ann = F, col = 'red')

> #Add the fitted data y-axis to the plot
> axis(4, las = 1, col = 'red')
```

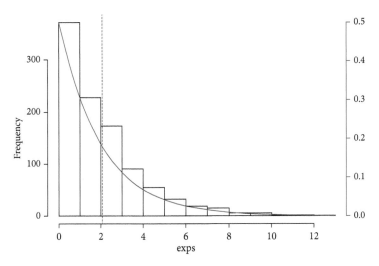

Figure 9.4 Our predicted distribution of coalescent events overlaid.

An exponential has a large variance: the square of the inverse of the rate parameter, which in this case is $(2N)^2$. We can integrate the distribution to find the point at which 95% of the coalescence events are likely to fall:

$$\int_0^x \frac{e^{-x/2N}}{2N} dx = 1 - e^{-x/2N}.$$

Substitute in 0.95 and solve for x:

$$0.95 = 1 - e^{-x/2N}$$

$$x = -2N \log{(1 - 0.95)} \approx 6N.$$

In other words, 95% of the coalescent events due to genetic drift of two lineages are expected to fall within $6N$ generations (in a population of constant size, etc.).

How about more than two lineages? If we add a third lineage, there are more opportunities for the first coalescence to occur, because there are more lineages in the population that can run into each other going backward through time in the genealogy. In fact, there are three ways to coalesce: A with B, B with C, or A with C. So the rate to the first event is three times faster:

$$P(x) = \frac{3}{2N}e^{-x3/2N}.$$

The average time until this occurs is the inverse rate or $(2/3)N$ generations. Then you are left with two lineages that take on average another $2N$ generations to coalesce:

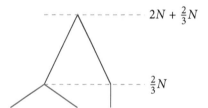

You can probably guess where this is going. With four lineages we have six ways to coalesce first, so the rate is $\frac{6}{2N}$ and the average time is $\frac{2N}{6}$ generations, at which point we are left with three lineages, ...

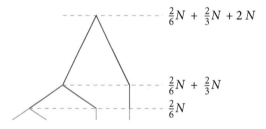

Here things start getting complicated in another way. There are two different *topologies* depending on which two lineages coalesce first and their relationship with the lineages that coalesce second. Compare the figure above (with a topology probability of 2/3) with the one below (with a probability of 1/3).

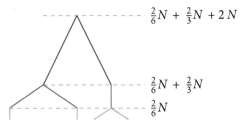

$$\tfrac{2}{6}N + \tfrac{2}{3}N + 2N$$

$$\tfrac{2}{6}N + \tfrac{2}{3}N$$

$$\tfrac{2}{6}N$$

Adding another sample can give us something like this (as an example among possibilities):

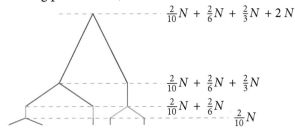

$$\tfrac{2}{10}N + \tfrac{2}{6}N + \tfrac{2}{3}N + 2N$$

$$\tfrac{2}{10}N + \tfrac{2}{6}N + \tfrac{2}{3}N$$

$$\tfrac{2}{10}N + \tfrac{2}{6}N$$

$$\tfrac{2}{10}N$$

... and here is a sixth sample ...

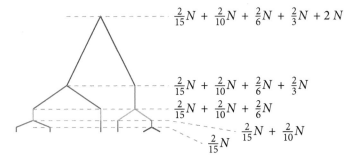

$$\tfrac{2}{15}N + \tfrac{2}{10}N + \tfrac{2}{6}N + \tfrac{2}{3}N + 2N$$

$$\tfrac{2}{15}N + \tfrac{2}{10}N + \tfrac{2}{6}N + \tfrac{2}{3}N$$

$$\tfrac{2}{15}N + \tfrac{2}{10}N + \tfrac{2}{6}N$$

$$\tfrac{2}{15}N + \tfrac{2}{10}N$$

$$\tfrac{2}{15}N$$

The expected time of each additional timestep between coalescent events follows the pattern

$$\frac{2N}{n(n-1)/2},$$

where n is the number of lineages that can coalesce at any given time. ($n(n-1)/2$ is the number of pairwise comparisons, also known as the triangular numbers.)

When the population size is large, we make a simplifying assumption that only bifurcations occur and only one coalescence event happens in each time period. You can start to see from these examples that increasing sample size tends to add short branches to the tips of the tree, not deep branches that reach back far into the genealogy. This (adding to the most recent tips rather than the interior) may seem strange, but realize that a small sample does not guarantee a connection through the deepest node; there is a small chance this is left out, and this is incorporated into the expectation. It can be shown, using inverse triangular numbers that form a telescoping infinite series, that the limit to this expectation with infinite sample size is only $4N$ generations back in time.

However, it is important to point out that this $4N$ is an expectation or average. There is a large variance in the times until the coalescence of all lineages and their effects on genetic variation. We are not going to get bogged down in the R code here, but, to point the way, consider simulating the coalescence of n lineages in exponentially distributed time steps, with Poisson-distributed numbers of mutations that get inherited to daughter lineages forward in time. To help you start exploring this, the function `coal()` is included in the *popgenr* package.

Imagine a change in the size of a population over time, such as a $10\times$ expansion or contraction. How might this affect the distribution of coalescent events across the genome? We will return to this question when we talk about tests of neutrality.

The concept of the coalescent can be used to derive some fundamental expectations in population genetics. It is helpful to realize that coalescence back in time is the same as genetic drift forward in time (coalescence to a common ancestor means that not all ancestral variation can be maintained in future populations). Consider drift-mutation equilibrium; what is the expected heterozygosity in a population? If each mutation generates a new allele at a locus (the infinite alleles model) the rate of mutation of pairs of lineages in each generation is 2μ. The rate of coalescence of pairs of lineages in each generation is $1/(2N)$. At equilibrium the average heterozygosity is expected to be the rate of mutation out of the total of both rates:

$$H_{IA} = \frac{2\mu}{1/2N + 2\mu} = \frac{2N}{2N}\frac{2\mu}{1/2N + 2\mu} = \frac{4N\mu}{1 + 4N\mu} = \frac{\theta}{1 + \theta},$$

where $\theta = 4N\mu$.

If we consider that on average two copies of a DNA sequence coalesce to a common ancestor $2N$ generations ago because the chance of coalescing in each generation is $1/(2N)$, then this is a total distance of $4N$ generations between the copies ($2N$ from one step back to the ancestor and then another $2N$ back down to the other copy). This gives a total of $4N\mu$ mutations on average between the two copies when we apply the per-generation mutation rate and assume that each mutation occurs at a new base-pair position in the DNA sequence (the infinite sites model). We get

$$H_{IS} = 4N\mu = \theta.$$

F_{ST} can be derived by considering the per-generation rate of coalescence of pairs of lineages as a fraction of the total rates of migration of lineages into a population, two pairs at a time, and drift:

$$F_{ST} = \frac{1/2N}{1/2N + 2m} = \frac{1}{1 + 4Nm},$$

where m is the per-generation migration fraction (and if you plot this you can see that only a small number of migrant individuals, Nm, in each generation can quickly homogenize populations).

Finally, the coalescent can be used to derive a common ancestry followed by an isolation model of F_{ST}:

$$F_{ST} = 1 - \frac{4}{4 + g/N},$$

where g represents the generations since isolation.

Curiously, if these two models (with very different assumptions) of F_{ST} are set equal to each other and simplified, we get $m = 1/g$. The coalescent has underscored that non-equilibrium shared ancestry with isolation and drift versus ongoing migration-drift equilibrium has inverse effects on expected F_{ST} and that F_{ST} alone cannot discriminate between them.

9.2 Tests of neutrality

Several tests of neutrality have been developed that are used to identify potential deviations from the model's assumptions. Here we will illustrate one influential test of neutrality, Tajima's D (Tajima 1989). Tajima's D works by comparing two estimates of $\theta = 4N\mu$ from a dataset. We have already derived θ_{IS}, equal to average pairwise heterozygosity, when we talked about the coalescent (also known as Tajima's estimator). There is an alternative derivation that can be made when considering the total number of alleles, or SNPs, in a collection of DNA sequences and the expected number of generations contained within the coalescent tree uniting them to a common ancestor. This is known as Watterson's estimator of θ or θ_W (Yong 2019). As we showed with the coalescent, the expected time to coalescence of n lineages is

$$\frac{2N}{n(n-1)/2} = \frac{4N}{n(n-1)}.$$

The sum of all coalescence times of a set of n initial lineages to a single ancestor is

$$\sum_{i=2}^{n} \frac{4N}{i(i-1)} = \sum_{i=1}^{n-1} \frac{4N}{i(i+1)}.$$

At each step between coalescence events there are $i + 1$ lineages (in the right-hand interpretation above) that can undergo mutations. So, when considering the number of alleles that can be generated over all lineages in a time period, we multiply by $i + 1$:

$$\sum_{i=1}^{n-1} \frac{4N(i+1)}{i(i+1)} = \sum_{i=1}^{n-1} \frac{4N}{i}.$$

We multiply the total time of all lineages in the tree by the per-generation mutation rate μ to get the total number of alleles we expect in a sample of n DNA sequences, and $4N$ is a constant, so we can place it outside of the sum

$$S = 4N\mu \sum_{i=1}^{n-1} \frac{1}{i},$$

where S is the number of SNPs in the collection of sequences.

This can be rearranged to estimate $\theta_W = 4N\mu$ from the number of SNPs:

$$\theta_W = \frac{S}{\sum_{i=1}^{n-1} \frac{1}{i}}.$$

Note that Watterson's estimator of θ requires an understanding of the coalescent of a set of lineages, but this was published in 1975 before the coalescence of more than two lineages was published (Kingman 1982).

Tajima's D is the difference between the average pairwise heterozygosity estimate of θ and θ estimated from the number of SNPs in a sample divided by the square root of the expected variance of this difference:

$$D = \frac{\theta_{IS} - \theta_W}{\sqrt{e_1 S + e_2 S(S-1)}},$$

where

$$e_1 = \frac{\frac{n+1}{3(n-1)} - \frac{1}{\sum_{i=1}^{n-1} \frac{1}{i}}}{\sum_{i=1}^{n-1} \frac{1}{i}}$$

and

$$e_2 = \frac{\frac{2(n^2+n+3)}{9n(n-1)} - \frac{n+2}{n\sum_{i=1}^{n-1}\frac{1}{i}} + \frac{\sum_{i=1}^{n-1}\frac{1}{i^2}}{\left(\sum_{i=1}^{n-1}\frac{1}{i}\right)^2}}{\left(\sum_{i=1}^{n-1}\frac{1}{i}\right)^2 + \sum_{i=1}^{n-1}\frac{1}{i^2}}.$$

This looks messy but the two different sums over n are found repeatedly in various positions and only need to be calculated once and then filled in.

This can be calculated with the following code (the average pairwise differences and S could also be calculated from a dataset, but we have left that out here for brevity):

```
> #Calculates Tajima's D
> theta_IS <- 2.8 # Average pairwise differences
> S <- 16 # Number of SNPs in the dataset
> n <- 20 # Number of allele copies sampled
>
> i1_sum <- 0.0
> for(i in 2:n-1){
    i1_sum <- i1_sum + 1/i
}

> theta_W <- S/i1_sum # Watterson's theta

> i2_sum <- 0.0
> for(i in 2:n-1){
    i2_sum <- i2_sum + 1/i^2
}

> e1 <- ((n+1)/(3*(n-1))-1/i1_sum)/i1_sum

> e2 <- (2*(n^2+n+3)/(9*n*(n-1))-(n+2)/(n*i1_sum)+
    i2_sum/i1_sum^2)/(i1_sum^2 + i2_sum)

> (D <- (theta_IS - theta_W)/sqrt(e1*S + e2*S*(S-1)))
[1] -1.409189
```

The first three variables would be adjusted depending on your data. In this example a $D = -1.409$ is returned. Informally, a D greater or less than two is considered significant; however, actual p-values are determined by simulation. Positive values of D indicate an excess of intermediate frequency alleles, which can be a result of a contracting population or balancing selection, since both of these extend the time of coalescent events in the older parts of a population's history. In a larger population there are more ancestors to choose from and coalescence is a rarer event, and inflates θ_{IS}, because older lineages tend to be shared among descendants at higher frequency relative to θ_W. This negative D indicates an excess of rare frequency alleles (the recent tips of the coalescent are magnified; they contribute more to S and θ_W than to average pairwise difference because they are rare), which indicates an expanding population, a selective sweep, or inefficient purifying selection against deleterious alleles. The key is to calculate D at a number of loci and look for outliers to flag putative selection candidates. Demographic effects like a change in population size should affect all loci in the genome, while selection is (generally considered to be) locus-specific in its effects.

There are a number of additional tests of neutrality, such as the HKA test (Hudson et al. 1987), the McDonald–Kreitman test (McDonald and Kreitman 1991), Fay and Wu's H (Fay and Wu 2000), and dN/dS ratios (Yang and Bielawski 2000). Many of these also utilize genetic changes that have occurred between species, and they all have their strengths and weaknesses. You are encouraged to explore these additional tests and learn about how they are used.

9.3 Linkage disequilibrium

A unique property of population genetics that is not found in similar fields such as evolutionary game theory is that alleles at different loci, or even different chromosomes, can be "linked" (although not always in the same sense as recombinant mapping in classical genetics) and inherited together more often than expected by random chance.

The degree of linkage disequilibrium (LD) is quantified by $\mathcal{D}$, not to be confused with Tajima's D. Consider two loci: one with an A/a polymorphism and another with a B/b polymorphism. We are curious about the association of alleles across loci that are inherited together. Using the multiplication rule of probability, we expect the frequency of AB haplotypes (p_{AB}) to be the product of the two allele frequencies $p_A p_B$ if they are inherited independently. The difference between these is quantified by $\mathcal{D}$ as a measure of linkage disequilibrium:

$$\mathcal{D} = p_{AB} - p_A p_B.$$

Depending on whether the *AB* haplotype is in excess or deficiency, $\mathcal{D}$ can either be positive or negative (or if you arbitrarily calculated $\mathcal{D}$ from the *ab* haplotype, the sign would change). $\mathcal{D}$ can also be calculated from all haplotype frequencies:

$$\mathcal{D} = p_{AB}p_{ab} - p_{Ab}p_{aB}.$$

To illustrate, let's say we have a small dataset of the following haplotype frequencies for two SNPs. One is an A/G polymorphism and the other has C/T alleles:

A-C 0.45

A-T 0.12

G-C 0.20

G-T 0.23.

Let's focus on the A-C haplotype. The frequency of the A allele is 0.57 and the frequency of the C allele is 0.65:

$$\mathcal{D} = p_{AB} - p_A p_B = 0.45 - 0.57 \times 0.65 = 0.0795$$
$$\mathcal{D} = p_{AB}p_{ab} - p_{Ab}p_{aB} = 0.45 \times 0.23 - 0.12 \times 0.20 = 0.0795.$$

Genetic drift, population structure, and strong selection are forces that can push $\mathcal{D}$ away from zero. There is a predicted exponential decay trajectory for $\mathcal{D}$ to return to zero over time in a large population, much like heterozygosity under genetic drift in a small population:

$$\mathcal{D}_g = \mathcal{D}_0(1 - r)^g \approx \mathcal{D}_0 \times e^{-rg},$$

where r is the recombinant fraction expected between the pair of loci of interest. This can be used to estimate the age of a haplotype. Finally, even for loci on different chromosomes that are independently assorting, $\mathcal{D}$ takes time to decay. Hardy–Weinberg genotypes can be restored in a single generation, but past events have lingering effects on LD, which can be used to infer processes further back in the past such as a population structure that no longer exists in the population.

When calculating $\mathcal{D}$ from actual datasets, the double heterozygotes are ambiguous. Say we have a C/T, A/G set of SNPs in an individual. Is the C allele associated with the A or the G allele at the second position? Often we don't know. But the frequency of haplotypes that are not ambiguous gives us information about the likely way to resolve double heterozygotes. If C-G haplotypes are very common and C-A haplotypes rare, then this suggests the C/T, A/G individual is likely to have C-G/T-A haplotypes.

Using this to calculate $\mathcal{D}$ is too cumbersome to work out by hand. Fortunately this is where the EM algorithm shines. Kalinowski and Hedrick (2001) worked with a bighorn sheep (*Ovis canadensis*) dataset (Boyce et al. 1997) to estimate LD. This species is rare and sample sizes are small, so we need to get as much information out of the data available as possible. The following R code implements the equations given in Kalinowski and Hedrick (2001). (The `Dcalc()` function is found in the *popgenr* package.) It starts off with a guess of equal haplotype frequencies and $\mathcal{D} = 0$. Then it updates this guess and quickly arrives at a maximum-likelihood solution of $\mathcal{D} \approx 0.0779$ and an a-B haplotype frequency of essentially zero:

```
> #Compound genotype frequencies
> AABB <- 2
> AaBB <- 0
> aaBB <- 0
> AABb <- 0
> AaBb <- 1 #Double heterozygote
> aaBb <- 0
> AAbb <- 1
> Aabb <- 0
> aabb <- 0

> #Run the function 'Dcalc' with the above inputs
> Dcalc(AABB, AaBB, aaBB, AABb, AaBb, aaBb, AAbb, Aabb, aabb)
```

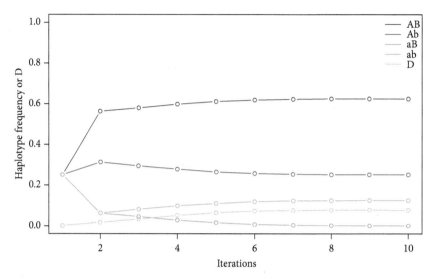

$\mathcal{D}$ is related to the statistical correlation coefficient (Pearson's) "r" that is used to measure linear correlations. Let's use $\mathcal{R}$ for the correlation coefficient to avoid confusing it with the recombinant fraction, r. $\mathcal{D}^2$ divided by the product of all the allele frequencies is equal to $\mathcal{R}^2$:

$$\mathcal{R}^2 = \frac{\mathcal{D}^2}{p_A p_B p_a p_b}.$$

In this case (which is easy to do directly on the R command line),

$$\mathcal{R}^2 = \frac{0.0779^2}{7/8 \times 5/8 \times 1/8 \times 3/8} \approx 0.237.$$

```
> 0.0779^2 / (7/8*5/8*1/8*3/8)
[1] 0.2367258
```

Also, strangely enough, if we multiply $\mathcal{R}^2$ by the total number of chromosomes sampled, which is usually $2n$ if we are looking at n diploid individuals, then we have a χ^2 statistic with one degree of freedom:

$$\chi^2 = 2n\mathcal{R}^2 = \frac{2n\mathcal{D}^2}{p_A p_B p_a p_b} = 1.89.$$

As we can see from R's built-in χ^2 distribution, this is not a significant level of LD.

```
> 1-pchisq(1.89, 1)
[1]  0.1692019
```

However, this should not be surprising. With sample sizes this small there is very little power to detect deviations, even if LD is very strong.

Finally we wish to point out that the EM algorithm is a "hill climbing" algorithm and finds a local maximum-likelihood peak. Other peaks are possible and MCMC methods can be used to deal with this and more fully explore complex-likelihood surfaces.

9.4 Deleterious alleles

Early in population genetics, deleterious alleles were not thought to have a significant population-wide effect at equilibrium, because it was assumed that deleterious mutations would be quickly removed by selection. Haldane (1937) realized that this was not the case, since there were many sites across the genome where deleterious mutations could occur, and negative selection would be frustratingly inefficient at removing all of them as they arose (JBS Haldane was also quite a character, look him up!). Haldane came up with the predicted equilibrium allele frequencies for deleterious alleles: $p \approx \mu/s$ for dominant phenotypes and $p \approx \sqrt{\mu/s}$ for recessive phenotypes. It is worth going through the derivation in his 1937 paper on your own.

He also came up with the idea of "genetic load": the average loss of fitness among individuals in a population due to deleterious alleles. Paradoxically, at equilibrium the average loss of fitness is not a function of the allele frequency or the strength of selection against the allele (these two factors counterbalance each other: a strong fitness loss will be maintained at a lower frequency and vice versa, so the average effect is the same). Rather, the loss of fitness and genetic load is only a function of the mutation rate. Increasing the mutation rate translates into a direct reduction in average fitness. This led to concern among geneticists about above-ground atomic bomb testing and increases in exposure to radiation in the Earth's atmosphere (not to mention exposure to chemical mutagens). When one extrapolates to the number of loci likely to be under purifying selection across the entire genome, it becomes clear that we can have a significant genetic load and that many species are not as fit as they theoretically could be in the absence of new mutations. Efforts to better understand this have led to a wide range of insights, such as the importance of recombination and likely fitness interactions (selective epistasis) among multiple loci.

There is not room to explore all of these ideas here, but we want to point out one important example. Deleterious mutations are constantly being removed from a population by selection. In the process linked neutral variation is also removed if it doesn't recombine away from the deleterious allele(s) to another haplotype background. This depression in neutral variation is predicted to be stronger in regions of lower recombination. This process and effect is known as background selection (Charlesworth et al. 1993; Hudson and Kaplan 1995). In essence, the effective population size, the amount of neutral variation that can be maintained, is not constant and changes along a genome depending on the fraction of copies that are not doomed for removal and cannot contribute to future generations. In fact, a correlation between genetic variation and rates of recombination has been observed for a number of species and is consistent with background selection (as well as hitch-hiking from selective sweeps; for example, Begun and Aquadro 1992; Innan and Stephan 2003). This effect, if not accounted for, can influence multilocus comparisons and contribute to false inferences of outliers (and positive selection) based on a range of measures such as θ estimates or F_{ST}, just to give two examples.

9.5 Fixation probability under selection and drift

Under selective neutrality the probability of occurrence of a mutant is the per-generation mutation rate (μ) times the number of allele copies that have the opportunity to mutate ($2N$). The probability of fixation of a new neutral mutation is equal to its starting frequency ($1/(2N)$). Thus the rate of neutral evolution, in terms of the fixation of changes along the lineage leading to a species, is $2N\mu \times 1/(2N) = \mu$; that is, the effects of population size cancel out and the rate of neutral evolution is equal to the mutation rate.

We can also talk about the rate of evolution of mutations under selection, both positive and negative. The general equation for the probability of fixation of an allele under selection is

$$\frac{1 - e^{-4Nsp}}{1 - e^{-4Ns}},$$

where p is the current allele frequency, s is the selection coefficient, and N is the population size (Kimura 1962).

In working with this equation some surprising results are found. For instance, the probability of fixation of a new adaptive mutation is only about $2s$. So if there were a 5% fitness advantage, the probability of fixation is only about 10%. Adaptive evolution is very inefficient! Most new adaptive alleles are lost due to drift when rare. We can combine this with the number of adaptive mutations expected in a population, $2N\mu_a \times 2s = 4Ns\mu_a$, where μ_a is the mutation rate that generates adaptive alleles, and see that the rate of adaptive evolution is a function of the population size—large populations can adapt faster than small populations.

This code plots the probability of fixation in a small population of $N = 100$ individuals when the allele starts as a new mutation, $p = 1/(2N)$, for a range of selection coefficients, s:

```
> N <- 100
> curve((1-exp(-2*x))/(1-exp(-4*N*x)), -0.01, 0.01,
        xlab="s", ylab="P(fixation)")
```

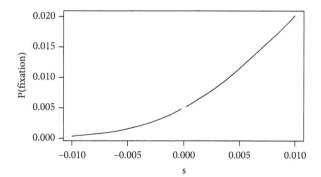

As $s = 0$ is approached, there is a region where selection is weak and the probability of fixation is close to the neutral fixation rate. This area is referred to as "nearly neutral." This gives adaptive alleles a slight boost in the probability of fixation. Unfortunately, it also gives deleterious alleles a probability of fixing. There is a chance of drift overriding selection and fixing an allele that causes a loss of fitness, which is more likely in small populations.

There are implications here for conservation genetics. Very small populations are inhibited in the rate of adaptation to keep up with disease and changing environmental challenges and are essentially irreversibly fixing deleterious alleles in the genome. It is useful to make some assumptions about the adaptive mutation rate, μ_a, and the much higher deleterious mutation rate, μ_d,[1] and predict the rate of adaptive and deleterious evolution[2] for very small populations such as the Javan rhinoceros (*Rhinoceros sondaicus*), with $N \approx 60$, compared to very large populations such as humans, with $N \approx 7.6 \times 10^9$.

One is tempted to say "nothing succeeds like success" in adaptive evolution; however, there are counterbalancing forces, as seen in these three examples.

1. Selective sweeps reduce flanking variation depending on the local recombination rate (a process known as hitch-hiking), which can reduce potentially adaptive genetic variation for selection to act upon, putting a slight break on things.
2. Larger populations have more opportunities for exposure to disease that can spread and lower population sizes, and may become a larger target for predators or parasites to evolve to exploit.
3. The evolution of selfish genes, which can lower fitness, is expected to increase with population size much like the adaptive evolution,

---

[1] Estimating μ_a is a subject of great interest. μ_d is perhaps on the order of 10^{-9} in humans and both are much smaller than the neutral mutation rate of $\mu_n \approx 10^{-8}$ per base pair per generation.

[2] A mutation must occur and fix, so multiply these together.

because they are both under positive selection; more about that in the next section.

9.6 Selfish genes

There are some genes or alleles of a gene that exploit biological tricks to increase in frequency despite having a fitness cost to the organism. These are known as selfish genes, and they underscore the fact that strong positive selection is not always equated with adaptation of the organism. There are a wide range of selfish genes with a range of dynamics—from "Medea" systems where the mother kills a fraction of offspring depending on their genotype (Beeman et al. 1992) to transposable elements that insert themselves across the genome and disrupt gene functions (for example, Nuzhdin and Petrov 2003 and references therein). However, here we briefly want to illustrate one well-known example, the mouse (*Mus musculus*) *t*-haplotype, that results in "meiotic drive" with a Bayesian approach to handling uncertainty in answering a question.

Approximately 90% of sperm from a male mouse that is heterozygous for a *t*-haplotype have the *t*-haplotype, contrary to the 50/50 expectation from a heterozygote. This is because the *t*-haplotype contains a "poison–antidote" system that is linked together in an inversion. The poison is exported to other sperm but the antidote remains behind in the sperm with the *t*-haplotype. Thus non-*t*-haplotype-carrying sperm are damaged, and the vast majority of offspring from a heterozygous male mouse will inherit the selfish allele. There are two important details that also need to be known. The *t*-haplotype results in a dominant visible phenotype; mice that carry it have shorter tails than normal and mice that are homozygous and carry two copies of the *t*-haplotype are essentially sterile.[3] Thus the *t*-haplotype cannot approach fixation because of negative selection against

---

[3] There are more complicated details than what is presented here; there are a range of haplotypes with a range of effects, but for now we are keeping the system simple; see Kelemen and Vicoso 2018 and references therein.

homozygotes, but can increase when very rare because of strong positive selection in the heterozygotes.

The t-haplotype is present at about a 10% frequency in wild populations of mice. You hypothesize that females avoid mating with t-haplotype-carrying males and you are interested in studying this—to do so you must estimate the frequency of different mating events. It is hard to observe mating directly, so you collect gravid females that are about to give birth. Say you have a gravid female that does not have the t-haplotype and make some simplifying assumptions such as that the female's offspring all have the same paternity and mating discrimination does not exist. What is the probability that the female mated with a t-haplotype-carrying male heterozygote?

Bayesian inference works with the intersection of the probabilities of models and data and is a way of working with uncertainty:

$$P(M_1|D) = \frac{P(D|M_1)}{P(D|M_1) + P(D|M_2)}P(M_1).$$

Here D indicates the data that is observed. M_1 is the model being considered (the father has a t-haplotype). M_2 is the alternative model (the father does not carry a t-haplotype). $P()$ is the probability of whatever is in the parentheses and | symbolizes "given." So on the left-hand side, $P(M_1|D)$ is the probability of the model given the data. On the right-hand side is the probability of the data given the model in the numerator with the probability of the model, $P(M_1)$, also known as the prior probability. In the denominator is the probability of the data integrated over all possible models. This could be written less formally as

$$P(\text{Model given the Data}) = \frac{P(\text{Data given the Model})}{P(\text{Data})}P(\text{Prior}),$$

and rearranging might give some insight:

$$P(\text{Model given the Data})P(\text{Data}) = P(\text{Data given the Model})P(\text{Model}).$$

Before observing any offspring, the prior probability that the female mated with a t-haplotype-carrying male, in the absence of mate choice effects, is $P(M_1) = 0.1$ because this is the frequency of heterozygous t-carrying males in the population. Say you observe a single offspring that develops with a normal-length tail. The probability of this under model 1 is 0.1 and the probability under model 2 is 100%. (Also note that we are looking at the probability of the data given one model as a fraction out of the total probabilities of the data of all models.) Now we can calculate the probability that the mother mated with a t male,

$$P(M_1|D) = \frac{0.1}{0.1 + 1}0.1 \approx 0.0091,$$

and the probability that the female mated with a normal male,

$$P(M_2|D) = \frac{1}{0.1 + 1}0.9 \approx 0.818.$$

So, even by observing a single offspring, it is much more likely that the father was not a t-haplotype carrier. Model 2 is approximately ninety times more likely than model 1. However, if even a single pup has a short tail the probability of M_2 becomes zero:

$$P(M_2|D) = \frac{0}{0.1 + 0}0.9 = 0.$$

9.7 Broadening the models

One of the most famous quotes in statistics is attributed to Dr. George Box: "All models are wrong, but some are useful."

In this book we have only considered variation of two or several alleles at one or two loci. While this has proven to be useful in understanding a wide range of naturally occurring genetic processes, many traits are influenced by genetic variation at a wide range of loci. This is an entire field of "quantitative genetics" and a lot of progress has been and continues to be made in expanding classical population genetics to encompass more complex models that will be useful in further understanding evolutionary genetics.

Also, population genetics perspectives are becoming more explicitly incorporated into other natural science disciplines such as ecology, where the focal unit (a population, a species, or a community) is generally assumed not to change rapidly over short periods of time—precisely what population genetics puts a lot of focus on.

9.8 R packages

One of the strengths of R is the ability to readily share novel functions and code through user-generated packages. At the time of writing, the Comprehensive R Archive Network (CRAN) has almost 16,000 packages available, and more besides are available as source code on various GitHub repositories and personal websites. Yet in this book we have not used a single R package besides our own *popgenr* package to load in data and provide a few key functions. This is not (solely) us being megalomaniacs who can't stand to share the accomplishments of others.

In composing this book, we consciously focused on building our exercises within the constraints of the default R environment, or "base" R. We did this because we believe that early understanding of the fundamental logic of the base R environment will provide the best foundational background to successfully implement any packages in the future. One notable family of packages we should mention is the `tidyverse` collection, which is formulated for data science in R. This collection includes packages such as `ggplot2`, `dplyr`, `tidyr`, and several others. These have all been designed with a consistent code formatting style, which at times can be quite distinct from a base R approach, and we heartily encourage new learners to familiarize themselves with it. You can install the whole suite of `tidyverse` packages by running

```
> install.packages(''tidyverse'')
```

Beyond the large number of functional statistics and data science focused R packages, there are a good number of R packages focused specifically on population genetics. Many of these include functions and datasets that directly help researchers to analyze real data. The number of packages that are actively maintained on CRAN can shift, but below we've compiled a non-comprehensive list of population genetics focused R packages that have been around for a while already, and have helpful documentation associated with them. There are so very many more packages out there, and we encourage you to explore the continuously evolving world of population genetics in R.

- *ape*—Analysis of Phylogenetics and Evolution. While focused on phylogenetics, the *ape* package provides many useful functions to calculate distance measures between genetic datasets.
  `http://ape-package.ird.fr/`
- *adgenet*—Exploratory Analysis of Genetic and Genomic Data. Extending the multivariate ecology data analysis package *ade4*, *adgenet* is built for the manipulation and analysis of genetic marker data and provides a good tool set for spatial genetic analysis.
  `https://github.com/thibautjombart/adegenet/wiki`
- *BEDASSLE*—Bayesian Estimation of Differentiation in Alleles by Spatial Structure and Local Ecology. A package aimed at quantifying the effects of geographic versus ecological distance on genetic differentiation. Provides a custom Markov Chain Monte Carlo (MCMC) algorithm to estimate the parameters of the inference model, as well as functions for performing MCMC diagnosis and assessing model adequacy. `https://cran.r-project.org/web/packages/BEDASSLE/index.html`

- *diveRsity*—A Comprehensive, General Purpose Population Genetics Analysis Package. Provides a variety of functions to calculate genetic diversity partition statistics, genetic differentiation statistics, and locus informativeness for ancestry assignment. Package is set up to provide for RAD-seq-derived SNP datasets containing thousands of marker loci. `https://cran.r-project.org/web/packages/diveRsity/index.html`

- *genepop*—Population Genetic Data Analysis Using Genepop. Provides the previously stand-alone program Genepop in R. Includes a series of functions and tools familiar to users of the Genepop sofware for processing and analyzing population-level genetic data. Documentation for the software is available at `https://kimura.univ-montp2.fr/~rousset/Genepop.htm`. `https://cran.r-project.org/web/packages/genepop/index.html`

- *hierfstat*—Estimation and Tests of Hierarchical F-Statistics. Provides multiple functions and flexible data formatting for estimating hierarchical F-statistics from haploid or diploid genetic data. `https://github.com/jgx65/hierfstat`

- *learnPopGen*—Population Genetic Simulations & Numerical Analysis. Conducts various numerical analyses and simulations in population genetics and evolutionary theory, primarily for the purpose of teaching (and learning about) key concepts in population and quantitative genetics and evolutionary theory. `https://rdrr.io/cran/learnPopGen/`

- *OutFLANK*—Population Genetic Simulations & Numerical Analysis. An F_{ST} outlier approach. Implements the method of using likelihood on a trimmed distribution of F_{ST} values to infer the distribution of F_{ST} for neutral markers. This distribution is then used to assign q-values to each locus to detect outliers that may be due to spatially heterogeneous selection. `https://github.com/whitlock/OutFLANK`

- *pcadapt*—Fast Principal Component Analysis for Outlier Detection. Methods to detect genetic markers involved in biological adaptation. Provides statistical tools for outlier detection based on Principal Component Analysis. `https://cran.r-project.org/web/packages/pcadapt/index.html`
- *pegas*—Population and Evolutionary Genetics Analysis System. Integrating well with both *ape* and *adgenet*, *pegas* provides an integrated modular approach for the manipulation of genetic data for population genetic analyses. `http://ape-package.ird.fr/pegas.html`
- *phytools*—Phylogenetic Tools for Comparative Biology (and Other Things). A wide range of functions for phylogenetic analysis. `https://github.com/liamrevell/phytools`
- *PopGenome*—An Efficient Swiss Army Knife for Population Genomic Analyses. Provides a suite of tools for population genomics data analysis in R. Optimized for speed via integration of C code. `https://cran.r-project.org/web/packages/PopGenome/index.html`

References

Allison, A. C. (1956). The sickle-cell and haemoglobin C genes in some African populations. *Annals of Human Genetics*, 21(1), 67–89.

Aminetzach, Y. T., J. M. Macpherson, and D. A. Petrov (2005). Pesticide resistance via transposition-mediated adaptive gene truncation in Drosophila. *Science*, 309(5735), 764–67.

Anonymous (2009). "Police Fear 'Serial Killer' Was Just DNA Contamination." Der Spiegel, March 26, 2009. Accessed XX XXXX. http://www.spiegel.de/international/germany/q-tip-off-police-fear-serial-killer-was-just-dna-contamination-a-615608.html

Attard, C. R., L. B. Beheregaray, K. C.S. Jenner, P. C.Gill, M. N.Jenner, M. G. Morrice, K. M. Robertson, and L. M. Möller (2012). Hybridization of Southern Hemisphere blue whale subspecies and a sympatric area off Antarctica: impacts of whaling or climate change? *Molecular Ecology*, 21(23), 5715–27. https://doi.org/10.1111/mec.12025 Data: https://doi.org/10.5061/dryad.8m0t6

Beeman, R. W., K. S. Friesen, and Denell (1992). Maternal-effect selfish genes in flour beetles. *Science*, 256(5053), 89–92.

Begun, D. J. and C. F. Aquadro (1992). Levels of naturally occurring DNA polymorphism correlate with recombination rates in *D. melanogaster*. *Nature*, 356, 519–20.

Boyce, W. M., P. W. Hedrick, N. E. Muggli-Cockett, S. Kalinowski, M. C. T. Penedo, and R. R. Ramey (1997). Genetic variation of major histocompatibility complex and microsatellite loci: a comparison in bighorn sheep. *Genetics*, 145(2), 421–33.

Buri, P. (1956). Gene frequency in small populations of mutant Drosophila. *Evolution*, 10, 367–402.

Chambers, J. (2014). Object-oriented programming, functional programming and R. *Statistical Science*, 29(2), 167–80. https://arxiv.org/pdf/1409.3531.pdf

Charlesworth, B., M. T. Morgan, and D. Charlesworth (1993). The effect of deleterious mutations on neutral molecular variation. *Genetics*, 134, 1289–303.

Clarke, C. A., F. M. Clarke, and D. F. Owen (1991). Natural selection and the scarlet tiger moth, *Panaxia dominula*: inconsistencies in the scoring of the heterozygote, f. *medionigra*. *Proceedings of the Royal Society of London. Series B: Biological Sciences*, 244(1311), 203–05.

Délye, C., M. Jasieniuk, and V. Le Corre, (2013). Deciphering the evolution of herbicide resistance in weeds. *Trends in Genetics*, 29(11), 649–58.

Edwards, A. W. F. (2008). G. H. Hardy (1908) and Hardy–Weinberg equilibrium. *Genetics*, 179(3), 1143–50. https://doi.org/10.1534/genetics.104.92940

Engels, W. R. (2009). Exact tests for Hardy–Weinberg proportions. *Genetics*, 183(4), 1431–41. https://doi.org/10.1534/genetics.109.108977

Fisher, R. A. (1922). On the dominance ratio. *Proceedings of the Royal Society of Edinburgh*, 42, 321–41.

Fisher, R. A. and E. B. Ford (1947). The spread of a gene in natural conditions in a colony of the moth *Panaxia dominula*, *Heredity*, 1, 143–74.

Gershberg, A., G. Neʼeman, and R. Ben-Shlomo (2016). Genetic structure of a naturally regenerating post-fire seedling population: *Pinus halepensis* as a case study. *Frontiers in Plant Science*, 7, 549. https://doi.org/10.3389/fpls.2016.00549 Data https://doi.org/10.5061/dryad.6r725

Gillespie, J. H. (2004). *Population Genetics: A Concise Guide* 2nd Edition, The Johns Hopkins University Press.

Graham, J., J. Curran and B. S. Weir (2000). Conditional genotypic probabilities for microsatellite loci. *Genetics*, 155(4), 1973–80.

Guo, S. and E. Thompson (1992). Performing the exact test of Hardy–Weinberg proportion for multiple alleles. *Biometrics*, 48(2), 361–72. https://doi.org/10.2307/2532296

Haldane, J. B. S. (1937). The effect of variation of fitness. *The American Naturalist*, 71(735), 337–49.

Hartl, D. L. and A. G. Clark (2006). *Principles of Population Genetics* 4th Edition, Sinauer Associates, Inc.

Hebert, P. D. and T. Crease (1983). Clonal diversity in populations of *Daphnia pulex* reproducing by obligate parthenogenesis. *Heredity*, 51(1), 353–69. https://doi.org/10.1038/hdy.1983.40

Hedrick, P. W. (2010). *Genetics of Populations* 4th Edition, Jones & Bartlett Learning.

Hornik, K. (2017). Frequently asked questions on R. https://cran.r-project.org/doc/FAQ/R-FAQ.html#Why-is-R-named-R_003f

Hudson, R. R., M. Kreitman, and M. Aguadé, (1987). A test of neutral molecular evolution based on nucleotide data. *Genetics*, 116(1), 153–59.

Hudson, R. R. and N. L. Kaplan (1995). Deleterious background selection with recombination. *Genetics*, 141, 1605–17.

Ihaka, R. (1998). R: Past and Future History. https://cran.r-project.org/doc/html/interface98-paper/paper.html

Innan, H. and W. Stephan (2003). Distinguishing the hitchhiking and background selection models. *Genetics*, 165, 2307–12.

Johnson, D. H. (1999). The insignificance of statistical significance testing. *The Journal of Wildlife Management*, 63(3), 763–72.

Kalinowski, S. T. and P. W. Hedrick (2001). Estimation of linkage disequilibrium for loci with multiple alleles: basic approach and an application using data from bighorn sheep. *Heredity*, 87(6), 698–708.

Kass, R. E. and Raftery (1995). Bayes factors. *Journal of the American Statistical Association*, 90(430), 773–95. https://doi.org/10.2307/2291091

Kelemen, R. K. and B. Vicoso (2018). Complex history and differentiation patterns of the t-haplotype, a mouse meiotic driver. *Genetics*, 208(1), 365–75.

Kimura, M. (1962). On the probability of fixation of mutant genes in a population. *Genetics*, 47, 713–19.

Kingman, J. F. C. (1982). On the genealogy of large populations. *Journal of Applied Probability*, 19, 27–43.

Lazarin, G. A., I. S. Haque, S. Nazareth, K. Iori, A. S. Patterson, J. L. Jacobson, J. R. Marshall et al. (2013). An empirical estimate of carrier frequencies for 400+ causal Mendelian variants: results from an ethnically diverse clinical sample of 23,453 individuals. *Genetics in Medicine*, 15(3), 178–86. https://doi.org/10.1038/gim.2012.114

Luzzatto, L. (2012). Sickle cell anaemia and malaria. *Mediterranean Journal of Hematology and Infectious Diseases*, 4(1), e2012065. https://doi.org/10.4084/MJHID.2012.065

Maryland v. King, 133 S. Ct. 1958, 569 U.S., 186 L. Ed. 2d 1 (2013). https://scholar.google.com/scholar_case?case=3234257148722545343

McDonald, J. H. and M. Kreitman (1991). Adaptive protein evolution at the *Adh* locus in *Drosophila*. *Nature*, 351(6328), 652–54.

Nei, M. and A. K. Roychoudhury (1974). Sampling variances of heterozygosity and genetic distance. *Genetics*, 76(2), 379–90. http://www.genetics.org/content/76/2/379.short

Nikolic, D., S. Cvjeticanin, I. Petronic, B. Jekic, R. Brdar, T. Damnjanovic, V. Bunjevacki, and N. Maksimonic (2010). Degree of genetic homozygosity and distribution of AB0 blood types among patients with spina bifida occulta and spina bifida aperta. *Archives of Medical Science*, 6(6), 854–59. doi:10.5114/aoms.2010.19291

Nuzhdin, S. V. and D. A. Petrov (2003). Transposable elements in clonal lineages: lethal hangover from sex. *Biological Journal of the Linnean Society*, 79(1), 33–41.

Paland, S., J. K. Colbourne, and M. Lynch (2005). Evolutionary history of contagious asexuality in *Daphnia pulex*. *Evolution*, 59(4), 800–13. https://doi.org/10.1554/04-421

Paul, D. B. (1995). *Controlling Human Heredity: 1865 to the Present*, Humanities Press.

Provine, W. B. (1971). *The Origins of Theoretical Population Genetics*, Chicago University Press, Chicago.

Purugganan, M. D. and D. Q. Fuller (2009). The nature of selection during plant domestication. *Nature*, 457(7231), 843–48.

Roewer, L. (2013). DNA fingerprinting in forensics: past, present, future. *Investigative Genetics*, 4(1), 22. https://doi.org/10.1186/2041-2223-4-22

Slatkin, M. and R. Nielsen (2013). *An Introduction to Population Genetics: Theory and Applications* 1st Edition, Sinauer Associates, Inc.

Stephens, J. C., J. A. Schneider, D. .A. Tanguay, J. Choi, T. Acharya, S. E. Stanley, R. Jiang et al. (2001). Haplotype variation and linkage disequilibrium in 313 human genes. *Science*, 293(5529), 489–93.

Taiwo, I. A., O. A. Oloyede, and A. O. & Dosumu (2011). Frequency of sickle cell genotype among the Yorubas in Lagos: implications for the level of awareness and genetic counseling for sickle cell disease in Nigeria. *Journal of Community Genetics*, 2(1), 13–18. https://doi.org/10.1007/s12687-010-0033-x

Tajima, F. (1989). Statistical method for testing the neutral mutation hypothesis by DNA polymorphism. *Genetics*, 123(3), 585–95.

Tian, X., B. L. Browning, and S. R. Browning (2019). Estimating the genome-wide mutation rate with three-way identity by descent. *The American Journal of Human Genetics*, 105(5), 883–93.

van't Hof, A. E., N. Edmonds, M. Dalíková, F. Marec, and I. J. Saccheri, I. J. (2011). Industrial melanism in British peppered moths has a singular and recent mutational origin. *Science*, 332(6032), 958–60.

Veale, A. J., O. J. Holland, R. A. McDonald, M. N. Clout, and D. M. Gleeson (2015). An invasive non-native mammal population conserves genetic diversity lost from its native range. *Molecular Ecology*, 24(9), 2156–63.

Waits, L. P., G. Luikart, and P. Taberlet (2001). Estimating the probability of identity among genotypes in natural populations: cautions and guidelines. *Molecular Ecology*, 10(1), 249–56.

Waples, R. S. (1989). Temporal variation in allele frequencies: testing the right hypothesis. *Evolution*, 43(6), 1236–51.

Weir, B. S. (1992). Population genetics in the forensic DNA debate. *Proceedings of the National Academy of Sciences*, 89(24), 11654–59.

Weir, B. S. (2012). Estimating F-statistics: a historical view. *Philosophy of Science*, 79(5), 637–43.

Wigginton, J. E., D. J. Cutler, and G. R. Abecasis (2005). A note on exact tests of Hardy–Weinberg equilibrium. *The American Journal of Human Genetics*, 76(5), 887–93. `https://doi.org/10.1086/429864`

Yang, Z. and J. P. Bielawski (2000). Statistical methods for detecting molecular adaptation. *Trends in Ecology & Evolution*, 15 (12), 496–503.

Yong, E. (2019). "The Women Who Contributed to Science but Were Buried in Footnotes." The Atlantic, February 11, 2019. Accessed xx xxxx. `https://www.theatlantic.com/science/archive/2019/02/womens-history-in-science-hidden-footnotes/582472/`

Index